Illustrated Guide to Aesthetic Botulinum Toxin Injections

Basics | Localization | Uses

A CIP record for this book is available from the British Library

ISBN: 978-1-85097-250-1

Addresses of the authors:

Dr. Michael Kane, MD
Kane Plastic Surgery
115 East 67th Street
New York City 10065
USA

Dr. med. Gerhard Sattler
Rosenpark Klinik
Heidelberger Landstr. 20
64297 Darmstadt
Germany

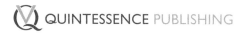

Quintessence Publishing Co, Ltd
Quintessence House
Grafton Road, New Malden, Surrey KT3 3AB
United Kingdom
www.quintpub.co.uk

Copyright © 2013 Quintessence Publishing Co, Ltd

Translated, revised and extended version (First edition)

Project management: Marie Bühler, Berlin
Photos: Peter Mertin, Marburg; Stephan Ziehen,
Hamburg; Marcus Karsten, Leipzig
Graphics: David Kühn, Berlin; Karl Wesker, Berlin
Typesetting: Kempken DTP-Service, Marburg
Production: Quintessenz Verlags-GmbH, Berlin
Printing: AZ Druck und Datentechnik GmbH, Berlin

Printed in Germany

Important note:

Like every other science, medicine is subject to constant development. Research and clinical experience widen our knowledge base, particularly with regard to medicines and other forms of treatment. If any dosages or methods of administration are mentioned in this book, the reader may have confidence that the authors, editors and publishers have taken great care to ensure that this information is in line with the latest knowledge available at the time of publication.

However, the publisher cannot give guarantees for any information regarding dosing instructions and methods of administration. All users are requested to take great care to check the package insert leaflets of the products used to establish whether the dosage recommendations or details of contraindications given therein differ in any way from the information given in this book. This sort of check is particularly important with rarely used or recently launched products. The use of any medication dose or method of administration takes place at the user's own risk. The author and publisher appeal to all users to inform them if they spot any obvious inaccuracies. The author and publisher are grateful for feedback of any kind.

Illustrated Guide to Aesthetic Botulinum Toxin Injections

Basics | Localization | Uses

Michael Kane, Gerhard Sattler

With 374 illustrations

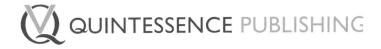

QUINTESSENCE PUBLISHING

London, Berlin, Chicago, Tokyo, Barcelona, Beijing, Istanbul, Milan, Moscow, New Delhi, Paris, Prague, São Paulo, Seoul, Singapore and Warsaw

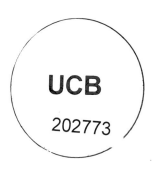

UCB

202773

Preface

For many years now, I have been focusing on aesthetic issues connected to aging. One of the procedures known for improving the visible effects of skin-aging is injecting botulinum toxin. While this procedure is common practice in Anglo-American countries in order to "smooth wrinkles," considerable skepticism can often be observed in European countries – e.g. Germany. Patients are often afraid of complications, side-effects, or even being poisoned. Also, many are distressed of the thought of establishing a mask-like, stiff appearance or others noticing that they underwent a botulinum toxin procedure. However, patients' anxiety regarding the procedure can be easily alleviated.

The real art of injecting botulinum toxin lies in selectively weakening muscle activity while considering the consequences on the entire appearance. This means that an intervention in the forehead area may also have an effects on the eyes and eyebrows. A consideration of the complex interplay between all mimic muscles is paramount. The most important precondition for a successful procedure is a sound knowledge of the anatomic topography of mimic facial muscles.

This is exactly where I see the focal point of this book: the reader will notice that the anatomical drawings are very precise. Of course those illustrations focus on an "average human," since every human is individually unique. Nevertheless, one can utilize the graphics in combination with the photographs and film sequences to display and understand functional connections. This comprehension, paired with an appropriate dosage, helps to virtually "model" the entire facial expression with botulinum toxin. The result is a youthful, alert, and healthy appearance. After the treatment, the patient is still able to express differentiated emotions while wrinkling in the treated area is considerably reduced. Moreover, the skin will be smoother and relaxed – a result of reduced tension within muscles connected to the facial skin. In addition to smoothing wrinkles, I observed that the entire skin of patients improved because of a homogenizing effect on the skin pattern and a reduction in pore size. These effects were particularly noticeable several weeks after the initial treatment. What is important to point out to the patients is that they should not be impatient when considering the desired results. Day by day they will be able to observe a gradual improvement in their appearance, as my photo documentation at the end of this book illustrates.

One note regarding dosage: all dosages and methods of treatment mentioned here are based on personal experience. I am very grateful that by gaining the support of my highly esteemed colleague, Dr. Michael Kane from New York, I was able to incorporate another opinion leader into this project. In order to calculate the ideal dosage, many important variables have to be considered: e.g. sex, age, basic muscle tone, muscle shape, and the extent of intended weakening of muscles, to name but a few. This list alone shows that the cited dosages are really only guideline values, which have to be adapted to the patients' needs. In cases of doubt, the treatment should commence with a weaker dosage and, if necessary, should be complemented with an additional injection after 14 days.

My intention was to create a practical workbook that offers a detailed overview of all the aspects of aesthetic botulinum toxin therapy. In particular, the chapters Organization and Documentation provide a good and specific outline of the entire practical procedure.

At this point I would like to thank all people involved in the development of this book, which is at the same time the cornerstone of a whole series. I am very grateful for the support of my family and the whole team of the Rosenparkklinik, especially my wife Sonja and my assistant Susanne Bernard.

Also I want to express my gratitude to my publishers Bernard Kolster and Marie Bühler who helped make a vision a reality and to the illustrator David Kühn, whose exquisite work deserves much praise. I owe particular thanks to Professor Fritz A. Anderhuber who supervised the anatomical drawings, and Professor Wolfgang Jost for reviewing the fundamentals chapter.

Finally I wish all the best to all colleagues and hope that this book will help in achieving positive therapy outcomes and our patients' satisfaction.

Yours,
Gerhard Sattler
Darmstadt, June 2013

Content

Abbreviations and symbols

The following abbreviations and symbols are used within this book:

ACh	Acetylcholine
BTX	Botulinum toxin
cm	centimeter
Da	Dalton
EMG	electromyogram
kDa	Kilodalton
ml	milliliter
mm	millimeter

SMAS	superficial musculo-aponeurotic system
SNAP-25	synaptosomal-associated protein of 25 kDa
SNARE	soluble N-ethylmaleimide-sensitive-factor attachment receptor
U	Units of biological activity
VAMP	vesicle associated membrane protein

⟶   Direction of motion

·················   Visualized auxiliary lines described within the text

● ○   Injection points

x   Orientation points

Link to video section and/or to website, enter accompanying URL or scan with your smartphone

1 The active substance botulinum toxin

1 The active substance botulinum toxin

1.1 Introduction

In its native form, botulinum toxin is a highly effective neurotoxin that inhibits signal conduction to the neuromuscular endplate. It is the most potent poison known to man and even miniscule amounts can be lethal. Its life-threatening dose of 0.001 mg per kg body weight is two million times lower than that of curare and a thousand times lower than that of diphtheria toxin.

Botulinum toxin is a metabolic product of the Gram-positive, spore-forming bacterium Clostridium botulinum. It is a ubiquitous bacterium, especially present in soil. The toxin in high doses can cause the disease known as botulism, a type of severe poisoning often acquired by consuming food that has become spoiled and contaminated with botulinum bacteria. The latency period to the onset of symptoms ranges from 4 to 6 hours, but may be up to 14 days in extreme cases. After an initial bout of gastroenteritis, followed by central nervous disturbances such as light flickering before the eyes, double vision, photophobia, difficulty swallowing and reduced salivary gland activity, the condition, if untreated, can lead to death due to respiratory paralysis.

However, increased understanding of the mechanisms of action of this neurotoxin has led to the therapeutic use of botulinum toxin in modern medicine. Apart from its use in the treatment of various neurological disorders, botulinum toxin has become established as the predominant treatment in aesthetic medicine. It is particularly widely used in the cosmetic reduction of wrinkles, achieved by inducing relaxation of overactive facial muscles.

1.2 Structure, serotypes

Botulinum toxin is a two-chain polypeptide consisting of a light chain (L-chain, approx. 50 kDa) and a heavy chain (H-chain, approx. 100 kDA), which are joined by a disulfide bond. While initially formed by Clostridium botulinum as a single chain, the toxin only becomes biologically active following enzymatic splitting (often called nicking) into the two-chain form by bacterial and eukaryotic endoproteases. The final active form of the protein is a complex make-up of the two-chain neurotoxin itself, together with hemagglutinins and non-toxin, non-hemagglutinin proteins. The hemagglutinins and the non-toxic proteins stabilize the neurotoxin and protect it from stomach acid when ingested.

Botulinum toxin can be divided into seven serologically distinct forms, types A to G. The amino acid sequences of the toxins have been decoded and show a high degree of homology to one another. Moreover, they show considerable similarities to tetanus toxin, also originating from a Clostridium species, which is why these substances are also jointly referred to as clostridial neurotoxins. The various serotypes differ in their duration of effect and potency, whereby type A has the most potent effect with the longest duration. Thus, type A shows an effect that is about ten times more potent than that of type C, while being as much as 50 times more potent than type B. Type A botulinum toxin is the main serotype in therapeutic use, especially with regard to aesthetic indications. Types B, C and F also play a role in therapeutic applications.

Molecular structure

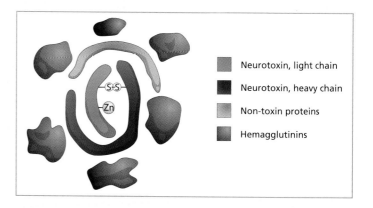

Schematic illustration of the biologically active botulinum toxin protein complex.

1.3 Mechanism of action

Botulinum toxin acts directly on the neuromuscular endplate and other cholinergic synapses, where it inhibits release of the neurotransmitter acetylcholine, leading to muscular paralysis of the affected fiber and loss of target organ function. The toxin's various serotypes all bind to the same receptor, but exert their effect on different proteins within cholinergic nerve endings. Three steps underlie the mechanism of action of botulinum toxin:

1. Binding
2. Internalization
3. Intracellular effect on SNARE proteins.

1.3.1 Binding

When the toxin is injected or absorbed from the gastrointestinal tract, its heavy H-chain initially binds to specific receptors on the plasma membrane of the cholinergic nerve endings. This binding to the presynaptic membrane shows a high degree of affinity and specificity.

1.3.2 Internalization

The neurotoxin is taken up into the nerve cell through receptor-mediated endocytosis. The heavy H-chain of the toxin allows the large molecule to penetrate the cell membrane and the endosome that is thus formed. The H-chain separates from the L-chain as the disulfide bond is broken. This allows the L-chain to enter the cytoplasm of the neuron.

1.3.3 Intracellular effect on SNARE proteins

The botulinum toxin light chain acts as a zinc-dependent endopeptidase with proteolytic activity. In the cytosol, depending on serotype, it splits a specific protein of the SNARE complex (soluble N-ethylmaleimide-sensitive factor attachment receptor), which is responsible for one step of the exocytosis of the acetylcholine vesicles. The SNARE

Physiological processes of neuromuscular innervation

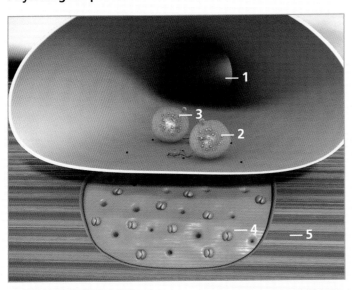

Overview – view into a synapse: As a result of a nerve stimulus, the synaptic vesicles, which contain the neurotransmitter fuse with the cell membrane. This causes the release of acetylcholine (ACh) into the synaptic cleft. ACh binds to the post-synaptic ACh receptors on the motor muscle cell. The depolarization triggered by this leads to contraction of the muscle fibers.

1 Synapse
2 Vesicle containing the transmitter
3 Acetylcholine within the vesicle
4 Acetylcholine receptor
5 Striated muscle.

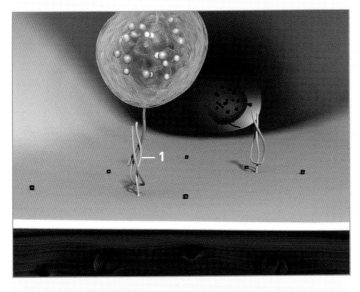

The release of ACh from the synapse takes place with the aid of a synaptic fusion complex, the SNARE complex. SNAP-25 and syntaxin are located on the cytosol side of the presynaptic membrane. They form a complex with the synaptobrevin, which is integrated into the vesicle membrane and anchors it to the internal neuron membrane.

1 SNARE complex.

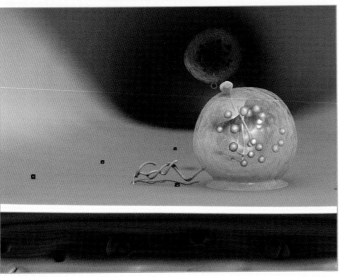

This three-protein complex initiates docking of the vesicle and its fusion with the presynaptic plasma membrane. Fusion leads to the release of ACh into the synaptic cleft.

1

The active substance botulinum toxin

Molecular mechanism of action of botulinum toxin A

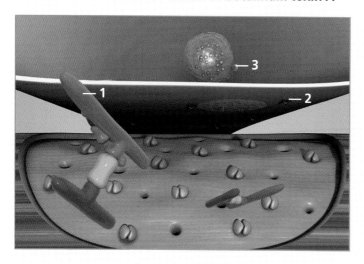

After the neurotoxin is injected into the muscle, it first binds to the ganglioside acceptor molecule (GT1b) with the carboxy-terminal domain of Its H-chain. A further receptor, the integral membrane protein SV2 (synaptic vesicle protein 2), is responsible for uptake of the toxin into the neuron. This receptor is accessible only after the release of acetylcholine into the synaptic cleft.
1 Heavy H-chain **2** Ganglioside acceptor molecule **3** SV2 receptor

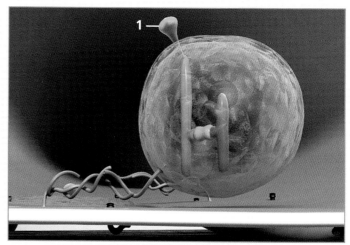

Botulinum toxin A, which has up to that point been fixed to the presynaptic cell membrane via the ganglioside bond, now binds with high affinity to SV2 and is taken up into the neuron by endocytosis.
1 SV2 receptor

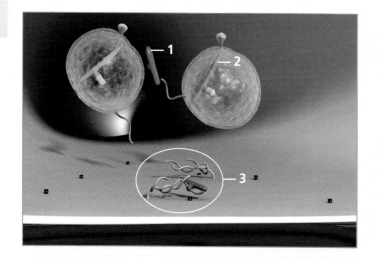

The contents of the vesicle are acidified by a protein pump. This changes the conformation of botulinum toxin A: the amino-terminal domain of the neurotoxin's heavy chain forms a pore in the vesicular membrane, the disulfide bridge is broken and the neurotoxin's light chain is extruded into the cytosol. The light chain of the botulinum toxin acts as a zinc-dependent endopeptidase, proteolytically cleaving SNAP-25 of the SNARE fusion complex and thus preventing the release of ACh into the synaptic cleft.
1 Light chain **2** Heavy chain **3** SNAP-25

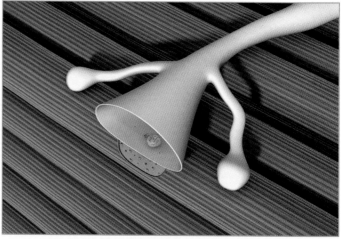

After that, the neurotoxin is broken down by proteases. The fusion protein SNAP-25, required for exocytosis, is formed again; the synapses regain their function after about 3 months. Once the synapse loses activity, neurite sprouting occurs by branching of the axon with the formation of new nerve endings. These gradually degenerate again following the synthesis of SNAP-25 in the denervated synapse and neuromuscular transmission is re-established.

complex is a fusion complex consisting of three proteins: synaptobrevin (also known as vesicle-associated membrane protein or VAMP), SNAP-25 (synaptosomal-associated protein of 25 kDa) and syntaxin. All three proteins are involved in the anchoring and thus the fusion of the acetylcholine vesicle with the plasma membrane. Inactivation of only one of these three proteins results in a non-functional fusion complex. Botulinum toxin types A and E attack and cleave SNAP-25. Types B, D, F and G split VAMP, whereas type C inactivates both SNAP-25 and syntaxin. By inactivating the SNARE complex, the botulinum toxins prevent the release of acetylcholine into the synaptic cleft. Stimulus conduction is thereby cut off. In striated muscle, this chemical denervation leads to flaccid paralysis, while in smooth muscle it produces atonia. The inhibition of sympathetic cholinergic nerve fibers causes a reduction or loss of sweating, referred to as hypo- or anhidrosis. The botulinum toxin effect described above can be put to therapeutic use in a variety of cosmetic and medical disorders.

1.4 Duration of effect

The main serotype used for the therapeutic applications of botulinum toxin is serotype A. Its initial effect sets in no earlier than 24 to 48 hours after the injection. Clinically relevant paralysis is observed after some 2 to 10 days. The peak effect is then reached after about 2 weeks. New SNARE complexes are formed 10 to 12 weeks after the injection. By this time, even the light chains of the toxin are inactivated and the nerve endings regain their original function. Thus, the effect of a botulinum toxin A injection persists for approximately 3 months. However, the clinical effect due to other factors including atrophy and behavior modification may last considerably longer.

Considerably longer efficacy periods have been observed in the treatment of hyperhidrosis. In these cases, remission has occurred after 6 to 12 months, and sometimes even after as many as 18 months. However, the causes of this have not yet been fully elucidated.

1.5 Products and dosage

For the majority of indications in botulinum toxin therapy, botulinum toxin serotype A is the most commonly used subtype. Medical preparations of botulinum toxin A are offered under a variety of trade names on the European and American market. However, the product offering remains manageable as it actually labels only a handful of individual substance preparations. At the publishing date of this manual, three manufacturer-specific preparations of botulinum toxin A are to be distinguished:
- IncobotulinumtoxinA (Merz Pharmaceuticals, Germany)
- OnabotulinumtoxinA (Allergan, USA)
- AbobotulinumtoxinA (Ipsen Biopharm, UK).

Product Name	Xeomin	Botox50/100 Botox50/100 Cosmetic	Dysport	Myobloc
Name of the preparation	Incobotulinumtoxin A	Onabotulinumtoxin A	Abobotulinumtoxin A	RimabotulinumtoxinB
Manufacturer	Merz Pharmaceuticals	Allergan	Ipsen Biopharm	Solstice Neurosciences, LLC
Botulinum toxin serotype	Type A	Type A	Type A	Type B
Active ingredient	Chlostridium botulinum toxin type A free from complex proteins	Chlostridium botulinum toxin type A	Chlostridium botulinum toxin type A	Chlostridium botulinum toxin type B
Units[1] per vial	50/100 U	50/100 U (Allergan units)	300/500 U (Speywood units)	5.000 U/ml
Inactive ingredients	Human albumin, sucrose	Human albumin, sodium chloride	Human serum albumin, lactose	Human serum albumin, sodium succinate, sodium chloride
Dosage form	Lyophilized powder in single-use vial	Vacuum-dried powder for reconstitution	Freeze-dried abobotulinumtoxinA	Clear and colorless to light-yellow sterile injectable solution
Reconstitution	Reconstitute vial with sterile, preservative-free 0.9% sodium chloride injection USP	Reconstitute vacuum-dried vial with sterile, non-preserved 0.9% sodium chloride injection USP	Each 300 Unit vial of DYSPORT is to be reconstituted with 0.6 ml of 0.9% sodium chloride injection USP (without preservative)	Ready to use; no reconstitution required; may be diluted with normal saline
Storage	Unopened vials: at room temperature 20 to 25°C (or refrigerator 2–8°C, or freezer -20 to -10°C), Reconstituted XEOMIN: 2–8°C, use within 24 h of reconstitution	Unopened vials: 2–8°C Reconstituted injection: 2–8°C, use within 24h of reconstitution	Unopened vials: refrigerated (2–8°C), protected from light. Reconstituted solution: refrigerate at 2–8°C, protected from light and use within 4 h	Store under refrigeration at 2–8°C, protect from shaking, freezing, and light. Diluted solution with saline: use within 4 h
Shelf-life	36 months	36 months	See expiration date	See expiration date
Indications	Improving the look of moderate to severe frown lines between the eyebrows (glabellar lines) in adults for a short period of time (temporary)	Improving the look of moderate to severe frown lines between the eyebrows (glabellar lines) in adults younger than 65 years of age for a short period of time (temporary)	Temporary improvement in the appearance of moderate to severe glabellar lines associated with procerus and corrugator muscle activity in adult patients <65 years of age	Treatment of adults with cervical dystonia (to reduce the severity of abnormal head position and neck pain)

1

The active substance botulinum toxin

Product Name	Xeomin	Botox50/100 Botox50/100 Cosmetic	Dysport	Myobloc
Remarks	The potency units of XEOMIN are specific to the preparation and assay method utilized, first effects within 7 days, storage at room temperature possible	LD_{50} units are specific for this preparation (Allergan units)	The potency units of DYSPORT (Speywood Units) are specific to the preparation and assay method utilized. They are not interchangeable with other preparations of botulinum toxin	Units of biological activity of MYOBLOC cannot be compared to or converted into units of any other botulinum toxin. Duration of effect in patients is between 12 and 16 weeks
Further information and supply	www.xeomin.com	www.botox.com	www.dysport.com	www.myobloc.com

Table 1.1 Overview of the FDA-approved botulinum toxin A and B products currently available on the market (June 2013). Provided product information is taken from the websites of the manufacturers. Besides the product names given above, there are further botulinum toxin products obtainable from various distributing companies that do indeed contain similar active substance preparations made by the same manufacturers. Products with identical substance preparations correspond with each other in their biological potency but can differ in the amount of active substance per vial and their approval regarding specific aesthetic indications.
[1] Units of biological activity (U) refer to preparation-specific median lethal doses (LD_{50}). The biological potency of one unit cannot be compared between products from different manufacturers.

The product names belongig to these preparations that have FDA-approval and are most familiar to international practitioners are (cf. also Table 1.1):
- Xeomin (IncobotulinumtoxinA, Merz Pharmaceutical)
- Botox (OnabotulinumtoxinA, Allergan)
- Dysport (AbobotulinumtoxinA, Ipsen Biopharm).

Along with these "big three," several further names of botulinum toxin A products are distributed on the market, in particular in Europe, by various companies. The ones that are recommend by the authors do indeed contain identical active substance preparations made by the same manufacturers as the products listed above. E.g. the company Galderma distributes in Europe the product Azzalure that contains the active substance similar to Dysport (AbobotulinumtoxinA), manufactured by Ipsen Biopharm as well. Products with identical botulinum toxin A preparations correspond with each other in their biological potency. But they can differ in the amount of active substance per vial and their approval status regarding certain indications managed by the regulatory authority of the respective country. E.g., Bocouture (IncobotulinumtoxinA, Merz Pharmaceutical), Vistabel (OnabotulinumtoxinA, Allergan) and Azzalure (AboboutlinumtoxinA, Ipsen Biopharm, distributed by Galderma) are the product equivalents to the trade names stated above, which are authorized for the treatment of glabellar lines in Germany. Whenever using a product for an indication not covered by the regulations of the responsible authority, patients have to give their consent to a so-called "off-label-use" (cf. section 1.12, p. 8).

The European counterpart to Myobloc is NeuroBloc (Eisai Co., United Kingdom). This botulinum toxin serotype B product is approved for the treatment of cervical dystonia by the Committee for Medicinal Products for Human Use (CHMP) of the European Medicines Agency. Further information respectively properties of the preparation, use and supply are to be found on the Web under:

http://www.medicines.org.uk/emc/medicine/20568

> The reader is kindly asked to check the prescribing information of the respective botulinum toxin product before usage and to visit the manufacturers' websites given in Table 1.1 in order to get any further information.

The biological activity of the serotype is the key determinant for the dosage of the individual products. The dosing recommendations are given in mouse units (MU) or units of biological activity (U) and relate to the biological potency of the respective products (1 MU = 1 U). One U corresponds to the amount of toxin, which kills 50% of a group of female Swiss Webster mice with a body weight of 18–20 g (LD50). The biological potency of one unit is specific to the preparation and cannot be equated amongst the products from different manufacturers. It is absolutely essential to take note of this when using the various products. The relative potency of the three commercially available botulinum toxin A preparations is a subject of great debate and of countless articles in the medical literature. Most clinicians regard the preparation of Allergan (Botox) and Merz (Xeomin) as having similar potency while the preparation of Ipsen (Dysport) is less potent per unit. As a guidance to the very inexperienced user, the authors describe an approximate dosage equivalence relation of 1 (Botox): 1 (Xeomin): 2.5 (Dysport), which means that an injection of 2.5 units Dysport and an injection of 1 unit Botox or Xeomin lead, as expected, to comparable clinical effects.

Correct administration of the active substance is a prerequisite for a successful treatment. The relevant information, such as anatomical and topographical landmarks, assessment of treatment outcome, doses, technique, and potential complications are described in the chapter "Regional Treatments" (cf. Chapter 5, p. 43 ff.).

1

1.6 Contraindications

Apart from hypersensitivity to botulinum toxin A, the contraindications include:

- Neuromuscular disorders such as myasthenia gravis, Lambert-Eaton-Rooke syndrome
- Allergy to the active substance or the additives
- Infection in the area being treated
- Coagulopathies
- Treatment with anticoagulants
- Drugs such as aminoglycoside antibiotics (gentamicin, spectinomycin, tobramycin, netilmicin, amikacin)
- Drugs with an effect on neuromuscular conduction (e.g. muscle relaxants of the tubocurarine type) may potentiate the effect
- It is the authors' opinion that botulinum toxin A should not be used during pregnancy or while actively breastfeeding, due to a lack of adequate data.

> **Cave**
> Botulinum toxin A should only be used with extreme caution and after careful consideration in patients with the above non-hypersensitivity contraindications.

Some relative contraindications include inflated expectations from the treatment by the patient and/or pathological distortions of body image (body dysmorphic disorder). These individuals show an excessive preoccupation with an imagined defect in their physical appearance.

1.7 Side effects

The use of botulinum toxin products is generally associated with few complications, but side effects can occur during treatment. The intramuscular or subcutaneous injection can cause pain locally. Swelling and reddening of the tissues can occur, as can local bruising. These complications can be magnified in patients who are anticoagulated or have coagulopathies. Contaminated injection sites can lead to infections. Allergic reactions have also been described. Side effects with a pharmacodynamic cause include excess weakening of the target musculature, as well as weakness of neighboring muscles. The extent and frequency of adverse effects vary considerably according to location, dose, injection volume and the type of product used. Like their desired effects, the undesirable effects of botulinum toxin products are typically reversible.

> **Further information on indications, contraindications, interactions and doses may be found in the relevant product monographs.**

1.8 Toxicity

The therapeutic range of the botulinum toxin products is very broad. While no human LD50-values are available, the lethal dose has been estimated at 200 ng, i.e. 5.000 MU Botox from trials with monkeys. This corresponds to about 50 ampoules. In therapeutic use, the highest recommended dose per injection session is needed in the treatment of spasticity of large muscles. It only rarely exceeds 400 MU Botox.

1.9 Systemic effect

Electrophysiological studies suggest that, when botulinum toxin products are injected, a small amount of the toxin reaches the circulation and exerts systemic effects. Thus, electromyogram (EMG) recordings have revealed changes in uninjected muscles far removed from the treatment site. In a few trials, investigation of the autonomic nervous system also showed slight changes in the cholinergic innervation.

A few of the side effects are attributable to this. Thus, systemic effects of the toxin may be responsible for mouth dryness and accommodation disorder – undesirable effects of treatment with botulinum toxin type B. Apart from this, however, most systemic effects are only detectable with extremely sensitive EMG equipment and are not clinically relevant.

1.10 Treatment failure

When botulinum toxin products are used, antibody formation may lead to treatment failure. Where this is the case, initially good treatment effects diminish following repeated injections. Botulinum toxin is a protein and can thus become a target structure for antibody production. The antibodies block the action of the toxin and may lead to permanent treatment failure. Potential risk factors for antibody formation include high doses and short intervals between injections. The low botulinum toxin doses used in cosmetic treatment mean that treatment failures due to antibody production are very rare. In contrast, treatment failures have been described in 2–5% of cases of cervical dystonia treatment with botulinum toxin type A; in more recent studies, however, this figure is now only about 1%.

Other serotypes, in this case types B, C and F, have been tested to provide affected patients with another treatment option. Serotype B showed the best effect in this context. Serotype F was also found to be successful in the treatment of parotid gland sialocele resistant to botulinum toxin type A. However, further studies showed that patients with immune resistance to type A botulinum toxin also usually develop treatment failure when treated with type B.

Various antibody screening tests can be used in everyday clinical practice to determine a patient's resistance status. In the "biological antibody test," a surface EMG of the extensor digitorum brevis muscle is used to record and document the amplitude of an action potential. The recording is repeated 4 weeks after the injection of a defined dose of the toxin and the amplitude compared with the baseline value. In patients who show antibody formation, the amplitude of the action potential remains unchanged. However, if the amplitude is reduced relative to baseline, a response to botulinum toxin type A is likely and the lack of therapeutic effect is attributable to other reasons (indication, choice of muscle, injection technique etc.).

1

To decrease the potential risk of treatment failure due to antibody production, the interval between treatment sessions should be as long as individual clinical judgment allows (the authors recommend a minimum of 2 months).

The antibody titer can fall after about 2 to 3 years, so a renewed treatment trial is advisable after this time.

1.11 Antidote

A polyvalent equine botulism antitoxin is available as an antidote to botulinum toxin. It forms part of the emergency supply at major hospitals and is used intravenously for the treatment of severe botulinum toxin poisoning. Even if it is often used too late to stop toxin that has already bound to neurons, the antidote can still neutralize any toxin circulating in the blood.

However, side effects that have already occurred after therapeutic use typically will not be remedied with the antidote.

1.12 Off-label use

The medical use of approved products outside the area stated by the FDA or by the regulatory authority of the respective country is referred to as off-label use. Like many other drugs, the various botulinum toxin products are also widely used for indications outside the approved area.

Apart from the treatment of disorders for which the botulinum toxin products have been approved, the use of these successful drugs has also become established for indications not covered by the product license. One of these areas of use is in the broad category of aesthetic medicine. The lines and wrinkles caused by facial expression can be smoothed with injections of botulinum toxin type A. The products Xeomin (Merz Pharmaceuticals, Germany) Botox (Allergan, USA) and Dysport (Ipsen Pharma, Germany; marketed by Medicis) are FDA-licensed for the treatment of glabellar lines in the USA. The treatment of other lines and wrinkles, and the use of these products for other cosmetic indications or in different countries are still classified as off-label use.

1

2 Documentation and organization

2 Documentation and organization

Documentation involves the collection of all the relevant patient data such as age, medical history, relevant concomitant illnesses, medication history and previous aesthetic treatments. All the treatments carried out are also recorded in the patient's file. Digital photo documentation provides a suitable before, during and after record of the treatment. A full consultation discussing the relevant risks and potential advantages of treatment needs to take place before any treatment takes place and must be documented by means of a written informed consent signed by the patient (cf. section 2.3, p. 17).

2.1 Photo documentation

Photography plays an important role in dermatology, plastic surgery, and aesthetic medicine as a simple and objective recording method. This section provides an outline of how documentation can be introduced into the practice and how the quality of photographic documentation may be optimized.

Busy, inhomogeneous backgrounds distract the eye from the subject

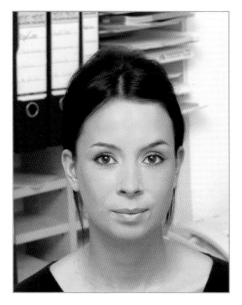 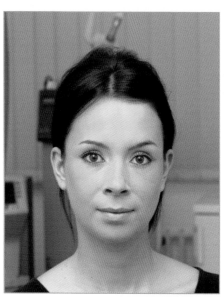 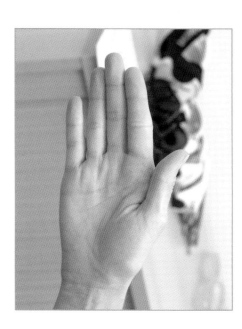

Office fittings in the picture.   Instruments in the background.   Dressings in the background.

Simple ways of improving the background

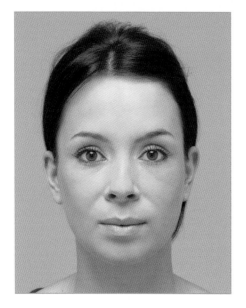 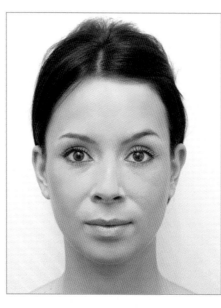 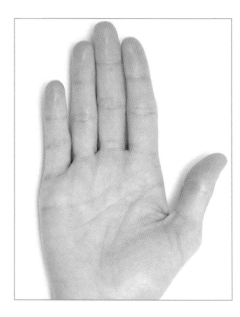

Door as background.   Room divider as background.   Examination couch as background.

2.1.1 Background

Ideally, photography should be performed in a dedicated space within the office. If a room of suitable dimensions can be reserved for photography, this will greatly assist in the taking of uniform photos. In this way, lighting, patient position, and distance to the camera can be controlled. Unfortunately, many offices do not contain the space for such a dedicated room.

Without such a dedicated space, there are still a number of things that can be done to standardize patient photographs. Ideally, the background should be free of extraneous objects that distract the eye from the subject, such as books, plants or other people. Furthermore, the patient being photographed for documentation purposes should not simply be placed into the middle of the room, as this makes the image background difficult to control, so that it is not easily reproduced for subsequent photos. The best way is to set up a fixed documentation spot within the practice premises, with a uniform, neutral background – e.g. a door, wall or room divider. E.g. good photographs of the head, arms, legs and feet can be taken against the neutral surface of an examination couch, so that no extraneous, distracting objects are visible in the background.

The ideal background is homogeneous in a single, neutral color. Colors that are too bright and glaring or too dark are best avoided.

Standard gray is useful when assessing skin changes. The background should be reproducible throughout the documentation period. At a minimum, a uniform flash and focal length (per body part photographed) should be used to minimize lighting and proportion differences.

> **Practice tip**
> Homogeneous areas in single color hues such as cream, light blue, or gray make a suitable background for photographic subjects.

2.1.2 Lighting

Every light source has different color temperatures, with differing effects on color reproduction. Artificial light sources pose particular problems, because mixtures of different light sources do not provide good follow-up documentation due to the color variations involved.

Mixed light situations (daylight, various fluorescent lamps or other artificial light sources such as incandescent bulbs) almost always occur in the practice setting, which makes it more difficult to reproduce the true colors of the subject and/or requires time-consuming post-processing with associated poorer quality.

2

Advantages and disadvantages of the direct flash

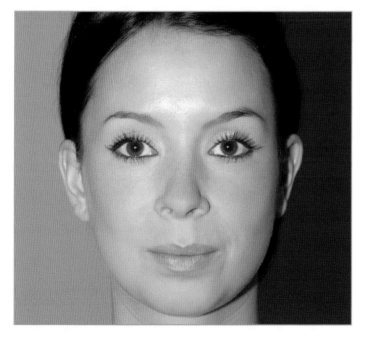

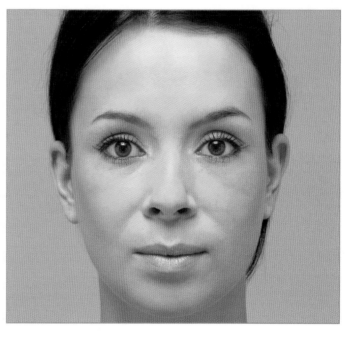

Direct flash
+ Contours are emphasized
+ Needs less powerful flash units
+ Easily controlled
+ Works with any flash
– Light distribution is not good
– Macro shots are difficult to achieve as the beam angle produces shadows at the lower margin of the shot
– The light diminishes rapidly, usually causing the tip of the nose, forehead and cheeks to appear lighter.

Indirect flash
+ Soft light
+ Uniform lighting
+ Light is distributed throughout the shot
+ Light does not diminish so rapidly
– Requires more powerful flash units
– The wall conditions need to be taken into account
– Requires experience

Effects of different light sources on the subject

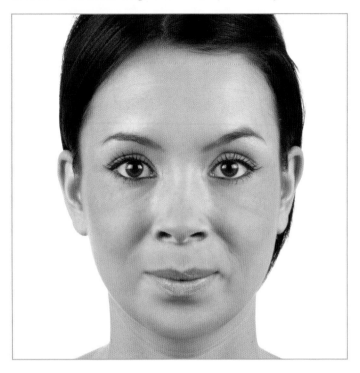

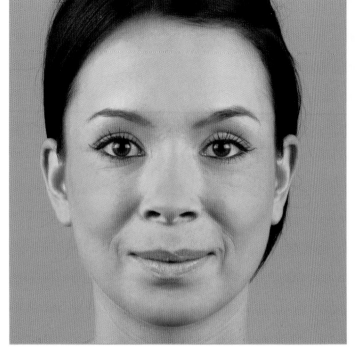

Light source: flash, set manually to cold light → color is falsified.

Light source: flash, set manually to incandescent flash → color is falsified.

Mixed light situations can be avoided by using a bright, artificial light source for the shots. The use of a dedicated flash unit is the optimal solution.

This allows reproducible results to be achieved regardless of daylight and also, in most cases, regardless of any existing ambient lighting. Exposure times suitable for excluding ambient light can be achieved with shorter shutter speeds from 1/125 s.

Lighting with a **flash** offers a few advantages, provided that the basic rules are followed. There are two variants: direct and indirect flash. For a direct flash, the adjustable reflector is directed at the subject. In the indirect technique, the reflector is directed onto a large white surface, e.g. the ceiling or wall of the room. The flash bounces off this surface, lighting the subject indirectly.

2.1.3 Camera

A choice of three camera types is available: compact (point-and-shoot), single lens reflex, or bridge cameras.

Compact cameras are all-round machines. They are small, easy to use, have an integrated flash and are suitable for simple documentation work.

The standard is a digital **reflex camera** with all its add-on options including lenses, flash, dermatoscope attachment or lens filters. If configured correctly, the digital reflex camera delivers the highest optical performance.

The other option consists of so-called **bridge cameras**. They combine the advantages of the digital reflex and point-and-shoot cameras in compact form.

Which of these three variants is selected depends on the user's individual requirements. In general, the selected camera should be suitable for its specialized use in medical documentation.

Practice tip
The camera should be tested before purchase. To do this, take long-distance and close-up shots of skin areas against single-color backgrounds. If the results are not reproducible, the camera's inbuilt features are not suitable for this purpose.
Before using a new camera, users should take time to familiarize themselves with its technical features and its operation.

Digital compact camera	Digital reflex camera	Bridge camera
Advantages		
+ Easy to use	+ Wide range of accessories available	+ Small and compact
+ Pre-programmed image modes	+ Simple manual operation	+ Can be operated manually
+ Economical to buy	+ High optical performance	
+ Small and compact	+ Lenses can be changed	
	+ Special attachments (e.g. dermatoscope)	
Disadvantages		
– Hardly any accessories	– Unwieldy	– Accessories expensive, few available
– Limited applications	– Basic knowledge of photography needed to operate it	– Lenses cannot be changed
– Manual operation complicated / few options		– Basic knowledge of photography needed to operate it
– No indirect flash possible		

Table 2.1 The camera types compared.

2.1.4 Taking photographs

The following section describes the basic practical features of photo documentation. The sample shots provided were taken with a digital reflex camera: after all the pros and cons are weighed, this type of camera is the most widely used documentation tool in dermatology, plastic surgery, and aesthetics.

Basics
For optimum results when taking photographs, the basic requirements include ensuring that the patient stands still in an appropriate pose, and that the camera is operated correctly. If a tripod is not used, the camera should be held close, with the photographer's elbow pressed tightly against the body to minimize camera motion.

Ensure that any measuring instruments and sensors are not covered with a finger or any other objects. They are there to ensure that the automatic lighting and focus functions work correctly.

The lenses and viewfinder should be cleaned regularly with cleaning agents designed specifically for the purpose. The sensor must not be either cleaned or touched. In essence, a defective sensor surface equals total damage to digital reflex camera.

The first or baseline shot of a documentation series should be taken carefully and conscientiously, as it represents the reference image. All the images taken during follow-up will be compared with this reference.

Detail shots
Before taking detail shots, it is often best to home in on the desired location gradually. If some time has passed since the last photo session, it can often be difficult to recall which area was last photographed. Where this is the case, a general view helps to find the correct location for subsequent shots.

Follow-up documentation
The reference photo is the baseline that is used when documenting a patient's follow-up course. This photo shows the selected distance, angle, light setting and location. These criteria are sufficient for most follow-up documentations. Higher-cost complete solutions (camera, tripod, light) are available for studies. With these, photographs can be taken under the same conditions.

Distance from the shot area
A certain distance needs to be maintained from the area being photographed, as the shot can otherwise become distorted or out of

2

Detail shots

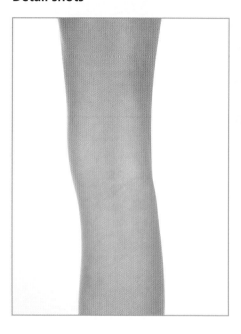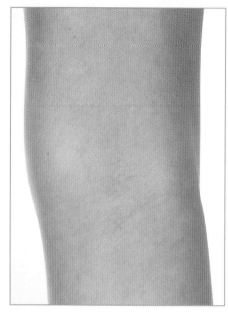

First take a general view and then zoom in on the area of interest in several stages.

Follow-up documentation: using the reference image as a guide

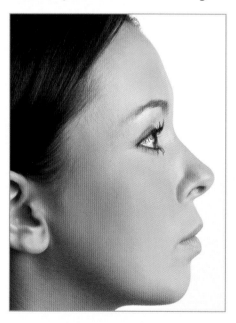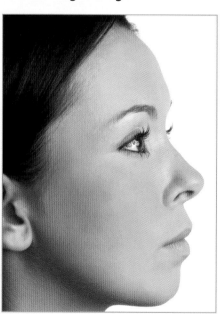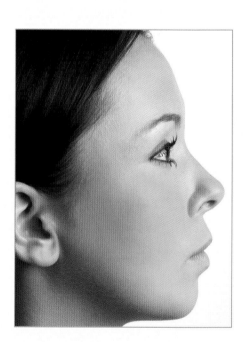

Reference image.   Follow-up image 1.   Follow-up image 2.

focus. Every focal length has its advantages and disadvantages in this respect. As examples, shots taken with a wide-angle lens of less than 50 mm can produce undesirable distortions (fish eye perspective) – rather like viewing someone through a spy-hole – which are not appropriate for most documentation purposes. These views can be of some use when photographing isolated lesions. It is better to zoom in on the subject from a slightly greater distance, as long as the focal length is consistent between photographs. On the other hand, one should also avoid zooming in too far, as this can cause blurring or changes in perspective.

Maintaining the correct distance from the area being photographed

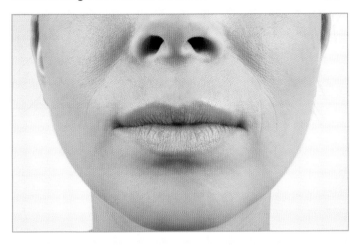 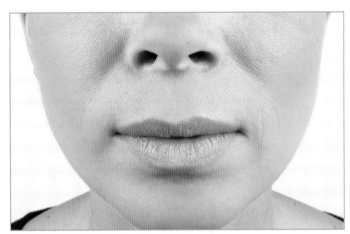

Distortions caused by moving the camera too close to the shot area.

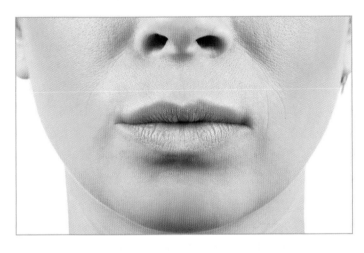 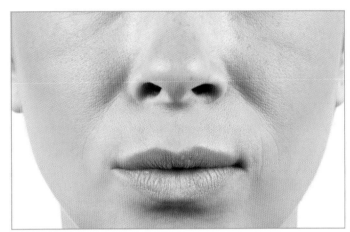

Better: shot taken by zooming in from a distance (100 mm focal length).

2

Correct camera angle

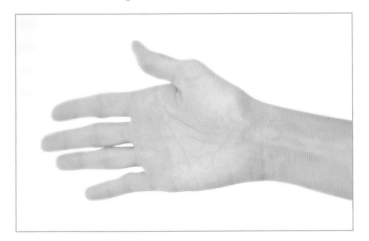 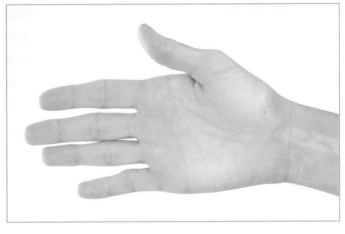

"Tipping" the camera causes some areas to be out of focus.

Ensuring that the camera is parallel to the imaging plane delivers sharply focused images.

Histogram and brightness levels

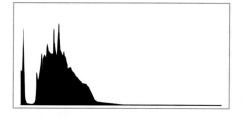

Underlit photograph.

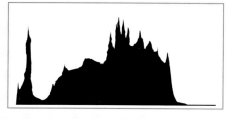

Normal lighting.

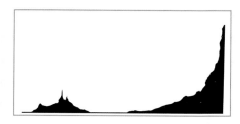

Overlit photograph.

Camera angle

The camera should always be held parallel to the subject, since standard cameras can only produce a sharply focused image in a plane parallel to the image sensor or camera. A partially blurred image is produced if the camera is tipped or tilted relative to the imaging plane.

Lighting

At best, assessing light through the camera display alone provides some guidance. An image that is too dark on the display indicates that there is too little light, a very light display indicates too much light. Different cameras (even those of the same type) can have different displays, and thus react differently to variations in lighting. The following parameters must be taken into account as regards lighting:

- ISO speed
- Lens aperture
- Flash unit performance.

The following settings are recommended: ISO speed over a range of 200–800, maximum possible lens aperture, an exposure time that fades out most of the ambient light when a flash is used, but which should not be longer than 1/50 s.

Measurement

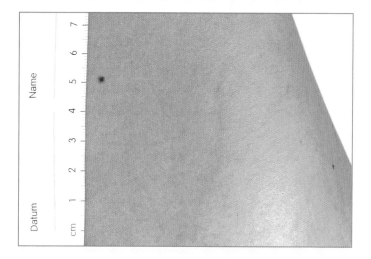

Self-adhesive disposable rulers can be used to document a dimension or a change during follow-up.

Uncertainties about correct lighting can be avoided by using a histogram. A histogram is a graphic representation of the brightness distribution within a photograph and provides a much better way of controlling this variable than the camera's own display. The two ends represent dark (left) and bright (right) areas in the image. However, a balanced, correctly lit photograph requires medium values in addition to the shadows and highlights. Depending on the camera model, the histogram can be displayed before or while taking shot, or it can be integrated into the playback mode after the shot is taken.

Measurement

The simplest way of making measurements in the image is with a ruler. If any features need to be documented with a "yardstick," a good option, for hygienic and practical reasons, is to use disposable rulers. These are usually 10 cm long and 2 cm wide, self-adhesive and can easily be written on with a ball-point pen.

2.1.5 Photo documentation checklists

Checklist: Fittings and equipment needed for follow-up documentation	
Background	• Wall 3 meters wide, in a single, muted color • Background system if appropriate
Camera	• Digital reflex camera, recent model • 10 to 15 megapixels • Low noise at high ISO speeds • Automatic sensor cleaning function recommended
Flash	• Dedicated flash unit made by the camera manufacturer • Adjustable reflector
Lenses	• 28 to 80-mm zoom lens, lowest aperture 5.6 • 100-mm macro lens, lowest aperture 5.6
Accessories	• Memory card • Card reader • Cleaning set for lenses and viewfinder • Bag

Checklist: Step-by-step photo documentation
1. Prepare room (darken, decide on a light source)
2. Select background (depending on location)
3. Select camera settings

4. Position patient, take general view photo followed by detail shots
5. For subsequent archiving: photograph patient's name or read the image into your database.

Checklist: basic camera settings	
ISO	No higher than 800
Focal length General view Details	35–50 mm 85–105 mm
Image format	JPEG; Fine
Compression	Medium compression
White balance	Set manually, adjusted to the light used
Exposure time	1/60 to 1/250
Aperture	5.6 to 11
Picture styles	Skin tones

2.2 Archiving

An archiving system is needed for case documentation. Data needs to be reliably stored and quickly retrieved. A variety of specialist systems exist for all areas of use. The following principles apply when archiving data:

- Regular backing up of data
- Making at least two copies
- Storing the copies in two different places.

2.2.1 Record sorting

The simplest way of archiving images is to store photographs on a magnetic data carrier such as a portable hard disk. Archiving on a CD or DVD is not advisable, as many optical media start to develop defects after only a few years and may become unreadable. Backing up of photographs and other data is also possible with many different secure web-based companies, which would protect your data in case of fire or other physical damage to the medical office.

Sorting should be based on the software used at the practice. One possible example would be to classify them by patient number and then by the date taken. In any case, plenty of thought is needed in advance when selecting the sorting method; otherwise, any subsequent changes in concept will necessitate changing all the data, to ensure the records can be properly tracked. The simplest way for your staff to sort photographs is in chronologic order.

2.2.2 Archiving using practice software

Many practice software manufacturers offer their own photo databases as part other patient data administration solutions. This image storing option can be very useful, as all the important patient data will also be available, and can be quickly retrieved with a targeted search.

2.3 Practice organization

It is well known that services such as the administration of botulinum toxin to treat the lines and wrinkles due to facial expressions are provided on a private, direct-payment basis. These services can and should be brought to the attention of patients. All staff members at the practice should also be familiar with the range of services available and be able to provide the relevant preliminary information regarding any individual supplementary services.

2.3.1 Appointment planning and information material

When planning appointments, an appropriate time slot will need to be allotted even at the initial enquiry stage. This is true even if a patient merely expresses an interest in, for example, a treatment with botulinum toxin. This time slot is important as it allows the patient's concerns to be explored comprehensively and professionally. The benefit of this time investment is that patients are fully informed, do not feel rushed, sold or has a greater potential for turning them into regular and satisfied patients. If patients at a practice are given all-round professional care, and if the treatment outcome meets the expectations of both parties, this sets up a solid and long-lasting patient relationship. Another aspect is that news of a cost-effective, very professional treatment with a good outcome tends to spread by word of mouth – representing the ideal form of practice growth.

This professional impression can be further enhanced by well-designed leaflets and brochures, displayed or handed out at the practice. This promotional material can be used to present and explain the individual procedures in a vivid and aesthetic format. Also, due to potential misconceptions the patient may have by reading misleading disinformation on the internet, these brochures can be used to educate your patients with proper information.

2.3.2 Information events

Well-informed and attentive practice employees, together with patient leaflets and brochures, provide one way of communicating what the practice has to offer. Another option is to hold presentation evenings on specific subjects. These can be advertised at the practice. Good promotional events, including case studies and treatment records, combined with a professionally delivered presentation, communicate competence and experience. These presentations also provide an opportunity for questions from interested parties to be answered, and for any misleading preconceptions to be either put into perspective or swept away altogether.

2.3.3 Waiting room TV

The waiting room TV set provides an additional channel of communication. Some suppliers provide very high-quality information for this medium. Some of the services on offer include short presentations, which give clear and informative depictions of various methods, such as wrinkle treatment options, and thus stimulate active enquiries. Of course, the other purpose of this medium is to introduce the practice team and the range of services provided.

2

2.4 The information session and informed consent

A treatment with botulinum toxin is preceded by a detailed **information session**, which is documented by means of a signed informed consent form. The person conducting the information session should:

- Provide an accurate explanation of the procedure
- Present the risks and side effects
- Describe the chances of success
- Clarify expectations and put them into perspective
- Inform the patient of alternative treatments, if any including no treatment
- Draw the patient's attention to the use of an off-label treatment, where appropriate
- Give a review of the medication guide/product insert warnings.

Simply handing out an information form does not replace the need for the information to be verbally imparted by a doctor. At the initial consultation, the doctor will often come up against certain prejudices and preconceptions, which need to be addressed. When being informed, the patient will often say that botulinum toxin injections utilize a dangerous poison that causes paralysis. This can be put into perspective by stating that the treatment proposed uses a drug and that the main aim of the treatment is not to cause paralysis, but temporary relaxation. At no time are the risks of treatment understated. The doctor and the team can also knowingly replace the term "paralysis" with more positive expressions.

During the information session, the patient needs to be questioned with regard to the following **contraindications**:

- Relevant previous illnesses
- Allergies
- Regular use of medication (particularly muscle relaxants, anti-coagulants, antibiotics)
- Possible pregnancy or breastfeeding.

It will also be valuable to know whether there have been any previous botulinum toxin treatments or other aesthetic procedures or operations to the face. Potential prior complications from these procedures should be noted. Active infection in the area to be treated represents a temporary contraindication.

Finally, the planned **procedure** and the next steps will need to be explained. The patient should have adequate time to consider the procedure and if unsure, encouraged to return home and think it over.

Another key point of the information session is to explain the **costs** of the treatment. Botulinum toxin is well known to be an extremely

Checklist: information session
1. The patient should to be informed about the chances of success, the relevant procedure-specific risks, treatment goals, the benefits to herself/himself, and the alternatives.
2. The less medically indicated, necessary or urgent the procedure, the more comprehensive the information weighing the risks and benefits should to be.
3. In a higher risk patient or procedure, the more comprehensive the information about unusual risks should be.
4. The more risky the side effects and interactions of a drug, the more comprehensively the patient will need to be informed about its risks. Information regarding medication that is not licensed for the indication in question (off-label use) is particularly significant in this context.

expensive active substance. These costs and the costs of the treatment will need to be met privately by the patient. A point to be taken account here is that a "wrinkle treatment" will need to be repeated after 3 to 4 months if the patient wishes to maintain their degree of improvement. The treatment fee will of course need to be individually discussed with the patient ahead of the procedure, ideally by the office staff. Clarity and transparency are important for the patient. In this respect, there should be clear price guidelines – either according to facial region or based on the units administered. Flat rates per administered unit can be charged when using botulinum toxin. This means that the costs are directly linked to the medication, providing a transparent charging mode. Likewise, flat rates per area treated can be charged, which may be easier for the patient to comprehend since it removes the concept of dosage from the fee. Each method has its advantages and disadvantages.

All the actions taken, from the information session/consultation and informed consent to the examination and the treatment, need to be **documented**. Special documentation forms, which can be kept in the patient's file may be useful for this purpose. Samples of these may be found in Chapter 7 (cf. "Aids for the Practitioner," p. 141 ff.), Aids for the Practitioner. Ideally, photographic follow-up documentation should also be carried out if possible. Any doctor who wants to use images of the patients for lectures or publications will need written consent from the patient for this purpose. An example of such a form that can be adapted may be found in Chapter 7 (cf. "Aids for the Practitioner," p. 141 ff.).

3 The examination

3 The examination

Conducting an examination or documenting the patient's baseline status forms the basis of a successful treatment. A more accurate and, most importantly, an individually tailored treatment plan can only be formulated once the patient's specific requirements have been evaluated.

Documentation plays an important role in this respect. Both the baseline examination findings and the measures taken are documented. The optimum approach – if this can be incorporated into the doctor's daily routine – is for the follow-up documentation to follow a fixed framework (e.g. before the injection, after the injection, eight days post injection, 20 days post injection). Special forms, as shown in Chapter 7 (cf. p. 142), are suitable for the treatment documentation. **Follow-up documentation** is greatly aided by the use of digital photographs, which should be taken under standardized conditions as far as possible (cf. section 2.1, p. 10 ff.).

Therapists should plan enough time for this, particularly if the patient is being treated for the first time. Therapists must also remember that a careful record of the baseline status is essential for precise therapy planning and that it justifies the time it takes. The following steps should be carried out in sequence:

1. History
2. Inspection
3. Palpation
4. Functional testing
5. Objective evaluation
6. Documentation.

These steps should be carried out in the stated order if a first treatment is involved. Apart from the purely organizational advantages of this sequence, it also gives the patient the confidence that the treatment will be optimally tailored to his or her needs – providing the foundation for a solid doctor–patient relationship, based on confidence and mutual understanding.

3.1 History

A broad general medical history is taken to elucidate the patient's general medical condition and to determine if the patient is a candidate for a non-essential aesthetic medical treatment. After this is done, the history focuses on the areas of dermatology, plastic surgery, and aesthetic medicine. In this context, it is just as important as the classical medical history, with which it has certain parallels. Points to be clarified are whether any aesthetic **treatments** have already taken place, what they were, when they were done, and how the patient rated their success. Prior complications from aesthetic procedures receive additional questioning and documentation. Particular areas of questioning include any previous surgical procedures to the face, such as blepharoplasty, brow lifts or facelifts. Special care is needed in these patients, due to the altered anatomical conditions. In this respect, the doctor must try to find out by history when any of these procedures were performed. Patients are sometimes reluctant to detail prior aesthetic surgical procedures.

In the classical history, the patient would report her symptoms. In the case of an aesthetic medical treatment with botulinum toxin, the history is more about her **desires**. In this case, therefore, taking a history leads not to a diagnosis, but to the specification and evaluation of the patient's expectations. Thus, unrealistic expectations that the patient has can be put into perspective during the history; in extreme cases, the patient may be advised against having the treatment.

Furthermore, the history should include targeted questions about a variety of aspects. These include the use of any **medication**, since certain drugs can have effects on the planned course of treatment with botulinum toxin A injections.

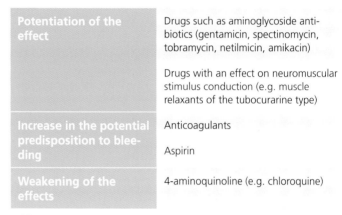

Potentiation of the effect	Drugs such as aminoglycoside antibiotics (gentamicin, spectinomycin, tobramycin, netilmicin, amikacin)
	Drugs with an effect on neuromuscular stimulus conduction (e.g. muscle relaxants of the tubocurarine type)
Increase in the potential predisposition to bleeding	Anticoagulants
	Aspirin
Weakening of the effects	4-aminoquinoline (e.g. chloroquine)

Table 3.1 Possible drug interactions with botulinum toxin A.

The patient should also be questioned about existing illnesses, which could also be of significance with respect to a planned treatment.

- Neuromuscular disorders such as myasthenia gravis, Lambert-Eaton-Rooke syndrome
- Allergies to the active substance or the excipients
- Infections in the treatment area
- Coagulopathies
- Botulinum toxin A is not recommended to be used during pregnancy and in nursing mothers due to a lack of adequate data.

The third complex that requires systematic evaluation is the patient's **lifestyle and environment**. She is asked about the nature of her work (especially prior to lower face treatment with toxin), dietary habits, the use of food supplements, smoking, the skincare products she uses, as well as exposure to sunlight.

3.2 Inspection

This also has a few parallels to the "classical" inspection. In this context, we should distinguish between direct and indirect inspection. In the indirect inspection, the patient is observed while behaving naturally, her facial expressions being noted while she is speaking, laughing and at rest. The direct inspection involves the targeted observation of individual actions such as frowning, raising the brows, smiling, and wrinkling the nose. These actions are observed both from the front and from the side.

3

Observation criteria for the frontal view

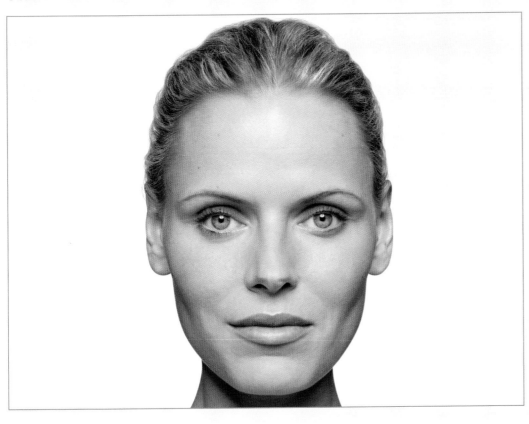

- Facial expression
- Assessing the wrinkles at rest
- Assessing the wrinkles under provocation
- Raising the brows
- Frowning
- Extreme smiling/closing the eyes
- Wrinkling the nose
- Turning down the mouth
- Facial symmetry.

3

Observation criteria for the side view

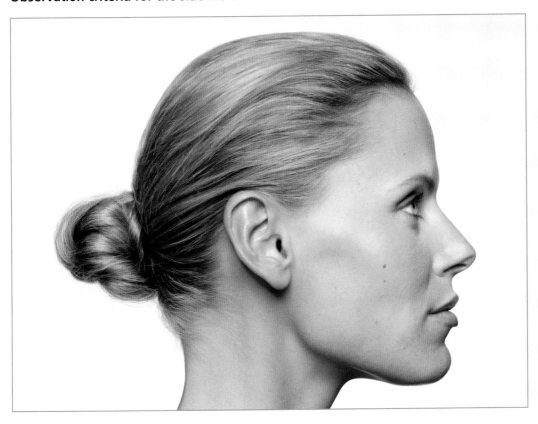

- Assessing the profile
- Assessing the state of the wrinkles at rest
- Assessing the state of the wrinkles under provocation
- Assessing the shape of the chin
- Protruding or receding chin
- Angle between chin and neck (double chin).

3.2.1 Skin color

Skin color changes with certain underlying disorders:
- Reddening can be a sign of a local inflammation, alcohol abuse, or a localized or generalized skin disorder.
- Bluish skin discoloration, due to a decreased hemoglobin or reduced oxygen level in the blood, may be seen in lung disease such as bronchial asthma or other disorders.
- Yellowish discoloration may be caused by liver disease or the use of certain food supplements, such as carotenoids.
- Brownish-yellow spots may occur in increased numbers during pregnancy and also with liver disease.

3.2.2 Skin condition

Various influences, such as the type of skincare (products) used, emotional circumstances or hormone balance, have an effect on the condition of the skin.
- In many cases, dry skin can be the result of over-intensive skincare. However, it can also be a sign of hypothyroidism, in which the skin of the face in particular appears thickened and rough.

- Autonomic reactions, such as may occur in anxiety or nervousness, can lead to increased skin moisture.
- Acne commonly develops on oily skin, particularly during times of hormonal change (puberty, menopause, treatment with hormone products).

3.2.3 Skin lesions

Efflorescences are frequently observed; they may be an indication of inflammatory skin disorders, which could represent a contraindication for injection treatment in the affected area.

3.2.4 Swellings

If unclear or postoperative swellings are detected in the patient's area of concern, the treatment should better be delayed until they have completely disappeared, since undesired dilution of the active substance and possible therapeutic failure could be the result.

3

Skin lesions

Macule: A macule is a circumscribed area of skin discoloration, which is smaller than 5 mm and is not accompanied by elevation, hardening or scaling. If the change is larger than 5 mm, it is sometimes referred to as a patch.

Squama: A scale is referred to as a squama. It consists of flat corneal cells that have become detached from the stratum corneum (horny layer).

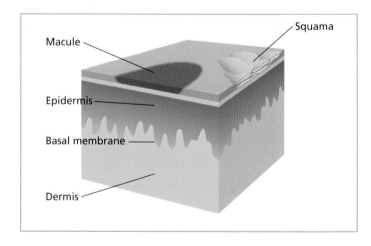

Papule: A papule is a circumscribed skin elevation that is smaller than 5 mm. If it is larger than 5 mm, it is referred to as a nodule.

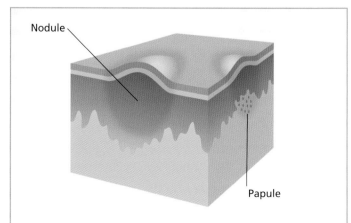

Bulla (blister): A hollow space filled with fluid is referred to as a bulla. If the lesion is smaller than 5 mm, it is more likely to be referred to as a vesicle or small blister.

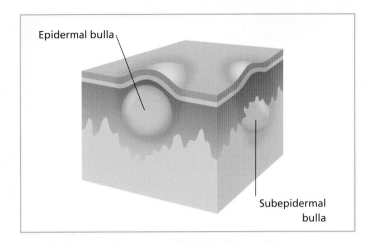

Pustule: A pustule is a hollow space filled with pus.

Wheal (urtica): A wheal is a transient, very itchy, usually pink plaque, formed as a result of edema in the dermis.

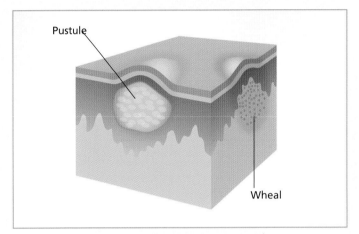

Erosion: An erosion is defined as the loss of epithelium (e.g. due to abrasion) down to the basal membrane. It heals without leaving a scar.

Excoriation: A change in the surface of the skin caused by scratching is called an excoriation. The tissue defect extends down to the stratum papillare (the papillary layer of the dermis).

Ulcer: An ulcer is a tissue defect that extends into the dermis or subcutis. It often heals with scarring.

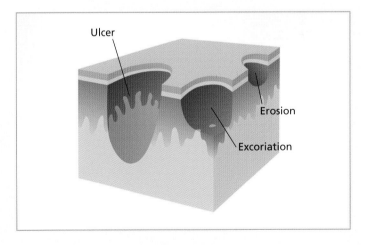

3

3.3 Palpation

Palpation represents another component of the assessment. Palpation of the skin comprises the qualities of temperature, surface consistency, turgor, and thickness. Turgor provides an indication of the fluid-dependent tensile state of the tissue. To assess it, a fold of skin is grasped between the thumb and index finger. When this skin fold is released, the skin normally snaps back smoothly straight away. If the fluid content is reduced, the skin fold remains in place or disappears slowly. Increased fluid or edema, especially in the peri-ocular area, is noted as well as this may become increased after treatment of the orbicularis oculi muscle.

Snap back test

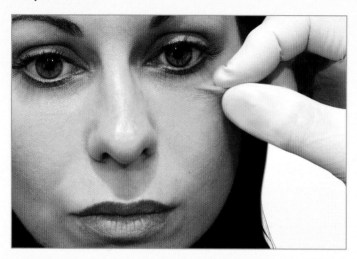 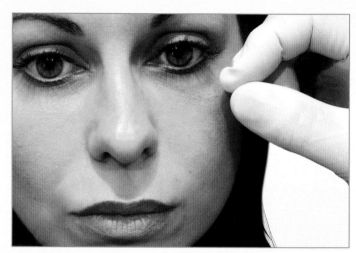

A fold of skin is grasped between thumb and index finger.

Normally, the skin snaps back smoothly straight away.

Bone prominences

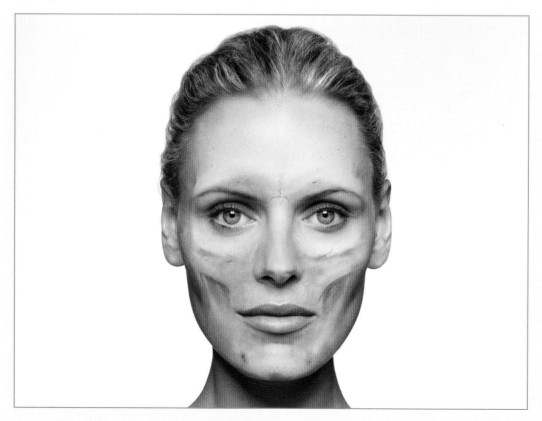

Overview of the palpable bone prominences.

3.3.1 Musculature

The superficial facial muscles radiate into the skin. It is difficult to differentiate between the individual muscles by palpation. However, palpation does make it possible to differentiate between increased or reduced muscle tone. The objective assessment of muscular activity is an important point in preoperative examination in order to chose an adequate dosage for the botulinum toxin injections (cf. Chapter 3.4, p. 25 f.).

3.3.2 Bones

The bony prominences palpable on the face, such as the upper and lateral orbital margin, the cheekbone, the mandible and the tip of the chin, provide an anatomical guide for the planned injections.

3.4 Functional testing

Besides the wrinkle severity evaluated during inspection, a functional testing of the involved mimic muscle is crucial for proper planning of treatment. Botulinum toxin A injections will lead to a dose-dependent attenuation of the muscle tone.

This is why the present state of muscular dynamics is determinant for an appropriate dose selection achieving natural wrinkle smoothing. Correct adjustment of toxin doses will prevent from overcorrection as well as from an undesired absence of the treatment outome.

A good way to assess the muscular activity involved in wrinkle formation is by palpating the patient's mimic areas in action. This is best done while asking him or her to perform various facial movements – e.g. raising the brows, frowning, closing the eyes tightly, wrinkling the nose or turning down the mouth. The Target of each investigation is the maximal muscular tension that the patient is able to produce while carrying out the facial action. To visualize examples for pos-

sible palpable findings, the authors decided to describe the muscle tones by the aid of amplitudes having peaks on a scale of 0–1.

From a clinical perspective, one can distinguish between three levels of activity: the first distinction that is made is between individuals with **hypokinetic** and **hyperkinetic movement types**. The former are characterized by less pronounced facial expressions. In contrast, those with hyperkinetic movements show active facial expressions and sometimes even exaggerated facial expressions.

The clinical relevance of this is that people with highly active, i.e. hyperkinetic muscle tone often need considerably higher doses. The dosing recommendations include a so-called correction factor to take account of this. In the end, this will come down to the therapist's instinct and experience with the treatment.

A further type, the **hypertonic type**, also needs to be included here from the clinical viewpoint. In this type, the muscles are constantly in a state of heightened tone, even though the individual in question is not aware of this. Repeated treatments at shorter intervals may be needed where this is the case. The patient should be told about this beforehand, to counter any unrealistic expectations of duration from the treatment.

As a general rule, the amount of muscular dynamic correlates with the age and gender of the patient. Men normally express more dynamic mimic activities than women, particularly with increasing age. The dose recommendations given in this manual mainly refer to women with intact moderate-toned muscle activities (~0.5). Depending on the patient's age and gender and, above all, depending on the individual findings after the functional testing, the practitioner has to consider possible dosage corrections.

Video: "Examination and functional testing"
http://www.kvm-tv.de/BTX/btx001.mp4

> Patients whose skin elasticity is preserved and whose facial expressions are active and dynamic, are typically the ones who benefit most from a course of treatment with botulinum toxin A. Patients with age-related loss of skin elasticity or those with skin changes due to intense and chronic exposure to the sun will usually have less impressive results. (Cf. fig. p. 26)

Illustration of mucle tones

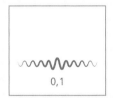
0,1

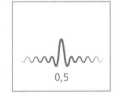
0,5

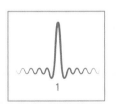
1

The illustrated amplitudes are representing muscular activities. Each peek shows the maximal amount of muscular tension that the patient is able to produce in conscious contraction of the mimic area. Patients with lower muscular activity (left) have to be treated with lower doses of botulinum toxin than people demonstrating enhanced muscular dynamic (right). The median amplitude represents moderate muscular dynamics commonly occuring in younger female patients.

> An objective evaluation of the muscular tensions involved in the formation of facial lines is elementary for an appropriate dosis selection in wrinkle therapy with botulinum toxin A. A patient with extraordinarily active mimic muscles has to be treated with higher substance doses to achieve the intended weakening. Hypokinetic patients with less pronounced facial expressions require lower doses, as overdosing can cause undesired rigidity.

3

Objective evaluation of wrinkles and muscle activities

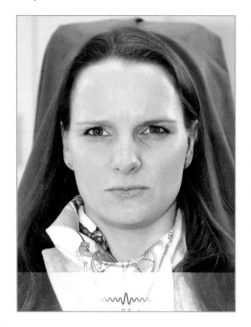 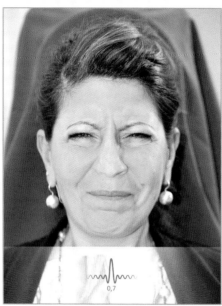 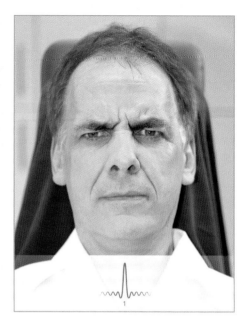

Gentle wrinkling at low muscle activity in the glabellar region (hypokinetic type).

Moderate wrinkling with higher muscular dynamic in the glabellar region (hyperkinetic type).

Deep wrinkling with exaggerated facial expressions and constantly heightened muscle tension in the glabellar region (hypertonic type).

3.5 Objective measures

Obtaining objective measures of the baseline findings provides the basis for treatment. When documenting the patient's chart, these objective measures also ascertain the effectiveness of the interventions carried. The purpose of objective evaluation is to monitor how the characteristics being evaluated have changed relative to baseline. Objective measures can be integrated into the documentation of the examination findings with little extra effort. Validated scales exist for evaluating the typical lines of facial expression; they are shown in Chapter 7 (cf. p. 142 ff.).

- Forehead lines (at rest and dynamic)
- Glabellar lines (at rest and dynamic)
- Brow positioning
- Lateral canthal lines (at rest and dynamic)
- Lip wrinkles (at rest and dynamic)
- Marionette lines
- Neck.

These scales allow both the baseline findings and the treatment outcome to be recorded, evaluated and objectively measured. Other scales or rating systems can be used as well. The key is that they are uniformly applied both before and after aesthetic interventions.

3.6 Documentation

In principle, the examination already forms part of the treatment – the part that precedes the therapeutic intervention. In practice, therefore, both the initial findings and the intervention must be documented. Chapter 7 (cf. p. 142), contains suitable documentation forms. All the relevant data can be recorded in this type of documentation form. Some electronic health record software systems have similar forms already integrated into the program. In addition to entering the patient's data and baseline findings, it is also used for entering the anatomical locations of the injection sites and the product used, with the following parameters:

- Units per injection site
- Total dose
- Reconstitution volume
- Batch number.

Treatment

4 Treatment

This section describes the relevant conditions to optimize the chances for successful treatment, ranging from the planning of treatment to the management of undesirable treatment effects. The following steps must be taken before treatment:

- Information session/consultation including evaluation of the patient's wishes (cf. section 2.3, p. 17)
- Obtaining an informed consent (cf. section 2.3, p. 17)
- Planning of treatment
- Examination with photographic documentation of the baseline findings at rest and with tensing of the muscles may also be useful (cf. section 2.1, p. 10 ff.).

The planning of treatment is guided by the wishes and needs of the patient. These are jointly established beforehand. In this context, the therapist may need to gently put into perspective any unrealistic expectations or results that cannot be achieved. To minimize miscommunication at the outset, the therapist should ask the patient to point out the region or regions that she would like to be treated and the issues that she perceives as problematic. A hand-held mirror is helpful for this. The patient can point out the details to the therapist directly using her reflection. The therapist can then also mark these details in directly with a marker (cf. section 4.4.3, p. 30), if desired. On the other hand, the therapist can also use the patient's reflection to explain the planned injection sites and treatment zones. The goals of wrinkle treatment with botulinum toxin A lie primarily in the reduction of the wrinkle depth in the region to be treated. Additionally, in good candidates, an improvement in facial shape can be achieved.

4.1 The treatment setting

The treatment setting and the atmosphere should communicate the maximum possible professionalism and care. A bright, well-ventilated treatment room set at a pleasant temperature helps achieve this. Ideally, the area being treated should be easily accessible from all sides to the therapist and any assistants.

The treatment itself should not be performed under any time pressure. Even with all the optimum preparatory consultations, the patient may still ask further questions, express concern or put forward additional therapy requests immediately before the treatment. The medical professional should react to these openly, patiently and without haste. An optimum treatment result is most likely to occur with full patient compliance. In this respect, it is advisable to describe the planned treatment in detail one more time. The actual treatment follows only after the outstanding questions have been answered and uncertainties laid to rest.

4.2 Positioning the patient

The treatment is usually carried out on a special treatment chair with adjustable height and reclining position. The working height is adjusted to the size of the therapist, to ensure that the work is done ergonomically, in an upright position and without straining the back. The back of the chair should be adjustable to allow it be smoothly lowe-

Treatment position

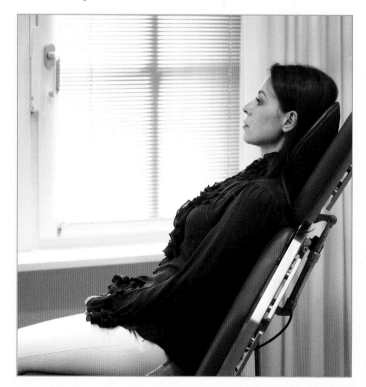

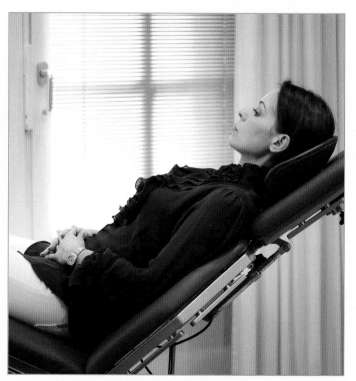

Upright position: Since the proportions of the face change with the patient's position, the planning of treatment takes place with the patient positioned upright.

Semi-supine position: The semi-supine position makes it easier for the patient to relax and allows the therapist to work more ergonomically, as all the areas of the face are easily accessible in this position.

red right down to a supine position. When doing so, it should be kept in mind that the proportions of the face in the supine position are different relative to the upright position. The planning of treatment on the face should therefore take place with the patient semi-supine or upright. Performing the treatment on a semi-supine patient allows her to relax more easily.

4.3 Ergonomics

In this context, ergonomics involves ensuring that the therapist can work in a posture that does not strain the back. An ergonomic posture without back strain allows him or her to carry out the treatment in a relaxed way, specifically aimed at avoiding back problems. Working with the upper body upright is one of the basic principles of an ergonomic posture. Twisting movements between the pelvis and pectoral girdle should be avoided. Any turning and postural changes should involve the whole body.

The treatment surface is at the optimal level if the treatment area is at the therapist's chest height. The therapist's shoulders can hang loosely and the injection arm can be supported by resting the elbow or forearm on the treatment chair. This allows a relaxed posture to be adopted when administering the injections.

4.4 Accessories

This section describes accessories that not only help optimize the therapist's technique, but also ensure that this almost painless therapy is even better tolerated by the patient. Needles and syringes are described in the next section (cf. section 4.5, p. 30 f.).

4.4.1 Topical local anesthetics

Local anesthetic creams may be applied before the treatment for particularly sensitive patients. One of the standard drugs is a combination of lidocaine and prilocaine (Emla). A mixture of lidocaine and tetracaine (Pliaglis) is also very effective. This gel acts rapidly with a very intense effect. For details of manufacturers, cf. Chapter 8, p. 167.

4.4.2 Loupe glasses

Loupe glasses enable the therapist to see stereoscopically when doing close work. Loupe glasses have a wide visual field and give a sharp, undistorted image even at the margins. Since the injections are administered with fine needles and relatively superficially, loupe glasses may be of benefit when doing this work. They allow the tiniest blood vessels to be identified and avoided, since blood vessels – particularly those around the eyes – can cause unsightly ecchymosis if traumatized during the injection.

4

Body posture during the treatment

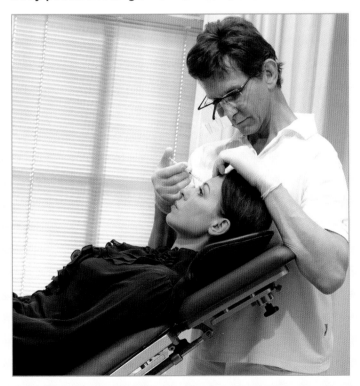

Optimal posture: In this posture, the therapist's pelvis and shoulders are not twisted relative to one another, the back is straight and upright and the injection arm is supported by the treatment chair.

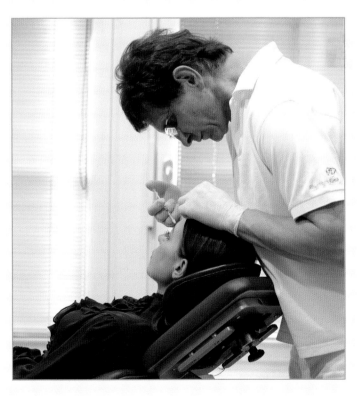

Incorrect posture: Here, the treatment surface is much too low: the therapist needs to bend his back, with increased strain on the cervical spine. This position does not allow the work to be done ergonomically and in a relaxed way.

4.4.3 Cosmetic pencil

An ordinary cosmetic pencil (eyebrow pencil or eyeliner) allows the injection areas to be marked before the treatment. This is also a good way of demonstrating the planned procedure to the patient.

The placement of these pencil marks is a matter for the therapist's personal preference. Many therapists do not mark in the injection sites beforehand, since the marks will need to be removed again when the skin is disinfected before the injection.

4.4.4 Coolpack

Coolpacks or ice cubes in plastic bags can be used before or after the treatment to relieve pain.

4.5 Syringes and needles

The injections should be administered as painlessly as possible. The correct choice of syringes and needles is an important factor in this respect. Insulin syringes represent the gold standard. They are used either with a very fine integrated needle or with a separate needle that can be fitted to the end. The therapist should hold the syringe in such a way as to ensure that he can read the graduations at all times, ensuring that the active substance is administered accurately and reproducibly. All the components of the syringes used should be latex-free.

4.5.1 The 0.3-ml syringe

These syringes are provided by various suppliers (cf. Chapter 8, p. 165 ff., for details of manufacturers). The needle has a diameter of 0.3 mm and is 8 mm in length. Due to the needle's special facetted

Treatment accessories

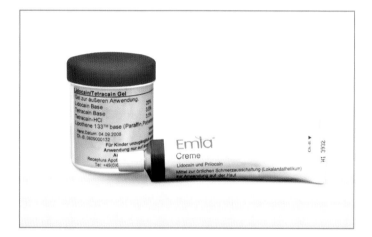

Topical local anesthetics: Lidocaine- or tetracaine-based local anesthetics can be used for anesthesia in sensitive patients.

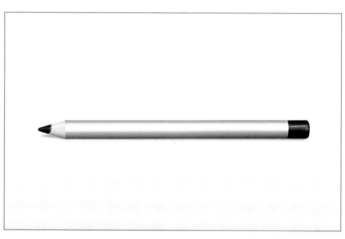

Cosmetic pencil: An ordinary eyeliner/cosmetic pencil can be used to mark the injection sites before the treatment and to discuss these sites with the patient if necessary.

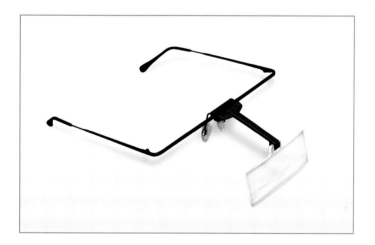

Loupe glasses: Loupe glasses like the ones shown here magnify the working area approximately four times and are an ergonomic aid to the therapist when administering the injections.

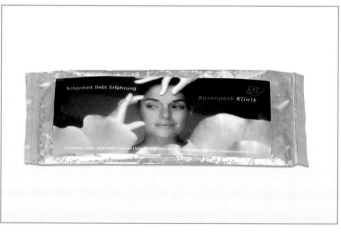

Coolpack: Coolpacks are suitable for both pre- and post-treatment. Coolpacks or ice cubes used before the treatment reduce sensitivity to pain. They also reduce swelling or pain if used after the treatment.

4

bevel, it causes very little pain when inserted into the skin. The needle's silicon coating also helps to minimize the pain felt by the patient. The syringe's clearly legible graduations allow precise dosing of the solutions being injected. Its design prevents a dead space, ensuring that the solution can be injected in full without any residue. A new syringe should be used after four to six injections. As these needles are very fine, they dull rather quickly with repeated skin puncture.

4.5.2 Single-use insulin syringe (1-ml volume)

The 1-ml syringe differs from the 0.3-ml version not only in volume, but particularly also in the fact that different needles can be fitted onto it. The volume of this syringe is 1 ml; its scale is divided into 0.1-ml graduations and is clearly legible. Minimal pressure on the plunger is needed for the injection, so that this type of syringe also enables the active substance to be dosed with ease.

4.5.3 Needles

Very fine needles, which are also intended for diabetics, are used to ensure that the injection is as painless and atraumatic as possible. The needles used in the injection treatment have a diameter of 0.25–0.30 mm and are 12–13 mm in length. The needles usually have a silicon coating, allowing them to penetrate readily and almost painlessly into skin and muscle. This is aided by the special facetted bevel of the needle tip. Most injectors use 30, 31, or 32 gauge needles.

4.6 Preparing the solution for injection

The active substance is initially supplied in powder form and must be reconstituted before the injection. This is best done using preservative-free, sterile normal saline (0.9% NaCl) solution. In the following section, the process for preparing a ready-to-use solution for injection is described using the product Xeomin as an example. The procedure is similar to that used for the products Botox and Dysport. The reconstituting instructions in the relevant product information texts should be referred to for further details.

Notes
- According to the package insert, the Botox 50 unit vials are diluted with 1.25 ml of preservative-free, sterile 0.9% NaCl solution.
- The Xeomin and Botox 100 unit vials are reconstituted with 2.5 ml of preservative-free, sterile 0.9% NaCl solution.
- Dysport 300 unit vials are reconstituted with 1.5 or 3.0 ml of preservative-free, sterile 0.9% NaCl solution.
- The units per milliliter ready-to-use solution of the three commercially available botulinum toxin A preparations can be read in table 4.1, p. 32.
- Many clinicians who are very experienced injectors use different reconstitution volumes than those above.
- Most clinicians also use preserved saline for reconstitution.

Syringe types

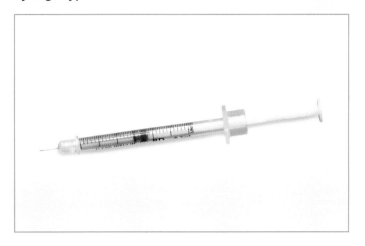

0.3-ml syringe with integrated needle: the volume of the syringe is 0.3 ml and there is no dead space. The clearly legible graduations allow optimal dosing.

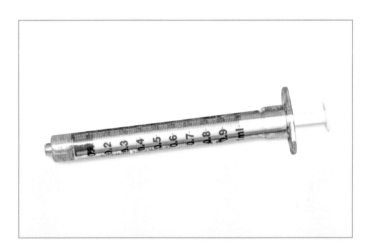

1-ml syringe: this syringe is used when administering larger volumes; precise dosing is made easy by the clearly legible scale and the low plunger pressure required to inject the solution.

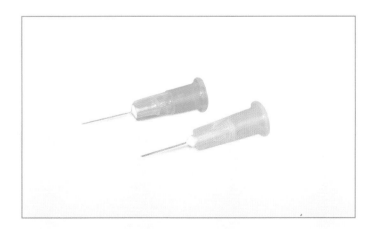

Needles: Very fine needles, also intended for diabetics, are used. They are 12–13 mm long and have a diameter of 0.25–0.3 mm (31 and 32 gauge). The silicon coating of the needles and the special bevel ensure that the injection causes little pain.

4

Treatment

The reconstitution of the vial contents and the withdrawal of the solution into the syringe should take place over a surface that is easily cleaned to catch any splashes. The exposed part of the vial rubber stopper should be cleaned with 70% alcohol before inserting the needle.

First, 2.5 ml of preservative-free, sterile saline solution is injected into the 100 unit Xeomin vial using a 2-ml syringe. The NaCl solution is drawn in directly by the negative pressure in the vial.

The vial is now carefully swirled until the substance has dissolved fully in the saline. Shaking must be avoided, as this generates foam; swirling prevents foaming. The ready-to-use solution can now be drawn up into suitable syringes (cf. section 4.5, p. 30 f.).

When drawing up the solution, care is needed to ensure that the tip of the needle does not touch the glass: this can damage the tip, making the injection painful for the patient. E.g. 1 ml of the reconstituted solution Xeomin contains 40 LD_{50} units. Therefore 0.1 ml of the solution contains 4 LD_{50} units (cf. Tables 4.1 and 4.2 for further details). According to the product insert, once reconstituted, the solution should be used within hours.

> The authors have taken all reasonable care in preparing the product information included in this book. They do not assume any liability or guarantee for the updated status, accuracy and completeness of the product information contained herein.
>
> Should the latest information or further explanation concerning the product reconstitution, use and safety of the products described in this publication be required, the reader is requested to read the FDA medication guides (cf. p. 154 ff) or contact the manufacturer or supplier directly.

Product	Units*/vial	Saline	Units per ml standard solution									
		ml	0.0125	0.025	0.05	0.075	0.1	0.2	0.3	0.4	0.8	1
Xeomin	100	2.5	0.5	1	2	3	4	8	12	16	32	40
Botox 50	50	1.25	0.5	1	2	3	4	8	12	16	32	40
Botox 100	100	2.5	0.5	1	2	3	4	8	12	16	32	40
Dysport 300	300	1.5	2.5	5	10	15	20	40	60	80	160	200
Dysport 300 (one-half dilution)	300	3	1.25	2.5	5	7.5	10	20	30	40	80	100
Dysport 500	500	1.5	2.5	5	10	15	20	40	60	80	160	200

Table 4.1 Units per ml ready-to-use solution after standard reconstitution. The information in this table refers to the 3 FDA-approved botulinum toxin A products in application for aesthetic indications (using 0.3-1 ml syringes). Figures do also apply to other product names containing identical substance preparations after similar reconstitution process.
* The biological potency of one unit is specific to the preparation and cannot be equated amongst products from different manufacturers.

Product	Ml standard solution	Ml saline	Units per ml "two-third dilution"					
		ml	0.01875	0.0375	0.75	0.15	0.225	0.3
Xeomin	0.1	0.2	0.25	0.5	1	2	3	4
Botox	0.1	0.2	0.25	0.5	1	2	3	4

Table 4.2 Units per ml ready-to-use solution after preparation of a "two-third dilution." The dilution adding two volumes of saline to one volume of the standard solution is useful in low-dosed injection of Xeomin or Botox when large diffusion is desired. The given information also applies to other product names containing identical substance preparations.

Preparing a "two-third dilution"

The "two-third dilution" is used by the senior author when he applies the preparations Xeomin or Botox where small doses together with a maximal diffusion range of the active substance are indicated (e.g. in lines on the forehead or fine wrinkles on the lower eyelid). To do this, 0.1 ml of the reconstituted standard solution is diluted with 0.2 ml of preservative-free, sterile 0.9% NaCl solution. This gives 4 units per 0.3 ml instead of 4 units per 0.1 ml as in the original solution (cf. Tables 4.1 and 4.2).

Preparing the ready-to-use solution

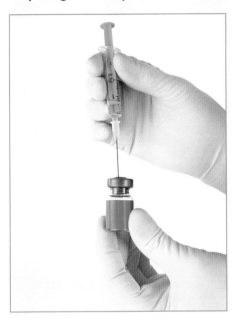

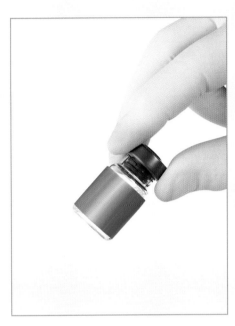

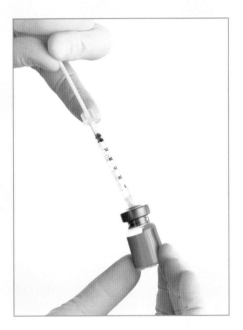

Step 1: Dissolve the active substance, supplied in powder form, with preservative-free, sterile 0.9% NaCl solution.

Step 2: Swirl the solution carefully until the active substance has dissolved completely. Caution: do not shake, as this causes foaming.

Step 3: Draw up the ready-to-use solution into suitable syringes.

4

4.7 Injection techniques

There are various injection techniques that can be used to administer the active substance. Five techniques are described below:

- Direct injection
- Two-level injection
- Intradermal wheal technique
- Directed injection
- EMG-guided injection.

Which technique is recommended in individual cases is dependent on the target muscle and the individual anatomical and functional findings in the target region as well as on the practioner's practical experiences. A general distinction is made between deep injections, which administer the substance directly into the muscle belly and superficial injections applying the substance in a subcutaneous level, from which it gets to its muscular destination gently via diffusion.

4.7.1 Basic rules

The practitioner may administer the injections either sitting or standing. In either case, care must be taken to work ergonomically (cf. Chapter 4.3, p. 29). The elbow of the injection arm should ideally be supported on the treatment chair or table. The syringe is held between the index and middle fingers, with the thumb placed loosely on the plunger. The injection hand is supported on the outer edge of the little finger either directly on the patient or on the non-injecting hand. This is the basic injecting position. Two fingers of the non-injecting hand can be used to fix and lightly compress the target muscle for a more precise injecting.

Video: "Basic hand position"
http://www.kvm-tv.de/BTX/btx003.mp4

The injection is carried out after provoked muscular activation. One of the basic rules is that the injections have to be as painless as possible for the patient. The use of syringes with extra fine cannula, as well as a careful insertion technique, are elementary in that context. Pain can be caused when the needle is inserted too deeply so that it pushes against the muscle-underlying periost and gets bent. To prevent this, needles always should be inserted slowly and diagonally to the skin surface.

Video: "Basic rules of injection"
http://www.kvm-tv.de/BTX/btx004.mp4

Tip

The senior author further recommends the so-called "knocking technique" to reduce pain during injection. By patting the patient's forehead with firm and rhythmical slaps, s/he creates mechanical deflection. In doing so immediately before the injection is done, the practitioner is able to decrease the injection pain by up to 80% as clinical experience has shown.

Treatment

General hand position

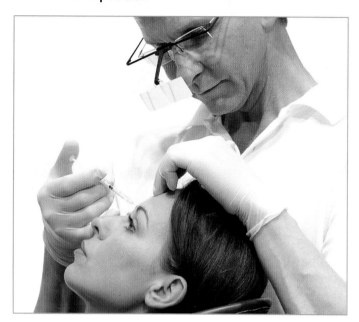

The syringe is held between the index and middle fingers, the thumb is placed loosely on the plunger and the injection hand is supported with the little finger. The needle should be inserted gently and in a diagonal direction to the skin surface.

Knocking technique

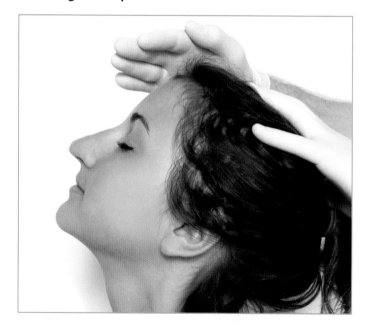

Rhythmical slapping on the patient's forehead before the injection is done will significantly reduce the pain during injection.

Besides prevention of pain, there are further basic rules important to follow during the injecting in order to avoid possible unwanted side effects of the therapy with botulinum toxin A. As an example, superficial subcutaneous injections or the use of dilutions (e.g. the "two-third dilution," p. 32) do allow an extra carefully substance dosing in areas with a given risk of overcorrection like the forehead. Concerning botulinum toxin injections around the eyebrows, a possible paralysis of the superior tarsal muscle (Mueller's muscle), leading to ptosis, has to be averted. Ptosis can occur after unwanted distribution of the substance behind the orbital septum, normally inhibited by the epicranial aponeurosis (Galea aponeurotica), which functions as a natural diffusion barrier. Along with careless injections, it is possible that the epicranial aponeurosis gets damaged by the needle allowing diffusion of the substance in the area of the superior tarsal muscle. For that reason, it is important to inject with a maximal distance to the orbital boundary. By using the thumb or forefinger of his contralateral hand, the practitioner is able to segregate the target muscle from its bony basis at a maximal level, ensuring safe injections along the eyebrow without the given risk of ptosis.

Basic rules for safe injecting

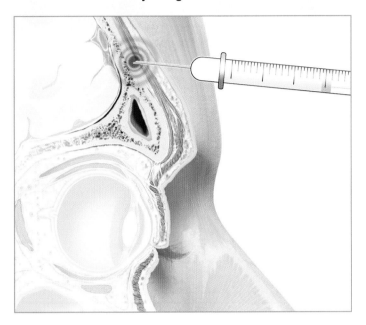

The fine needles used for botulinum toxin injections can bend if they reach the periost, which will cause pain while performing injections. For that reason, injections to the bone have to be avoided in any case.

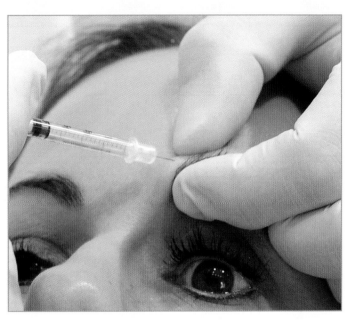

By carefully inserting the needle in a diagonal direction to the skin surface, injections are as painless as possible.

4

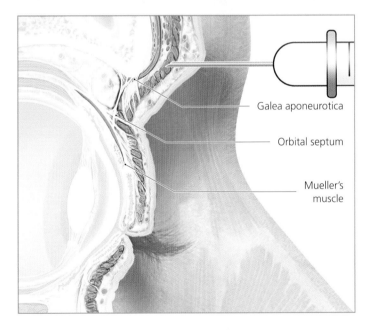

Galea aponeurotica

Orbital septum

Mueller's muscle

When injecting near the eyebrow, possible windowing of the epicranial aponeurosis by the needle can lead to an undesired diffusion of the active substance behind the orbital septum causing paralysis of the Mueller's muscle and ptosis.

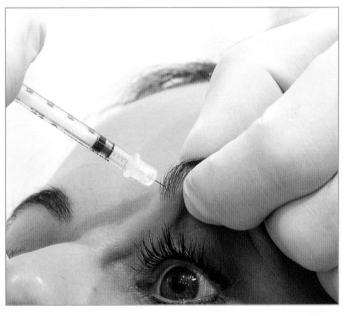

Two fingers of the non-injecting hand are used to create a maximal distance between the muscular target parts and the orbital margin, allowing safe injecting.

Video: "Rules for safe injecting"
http://www.kvm-tv.de/BTX/btx005.mp4

4.7.2 Direct injection

For the direct injection, the needle is inserted perpendicularly to the skin. The botulinum toxin is injected into the belly of the target muscle, located beforehand by palpation. To ensure more accurate placement of the drug, the muscle can also be held in place between the thumb and index finger of the free hand and compressed lightly.

Video: "Direct Injection technique"
http://www.kvm-tv.de/BTX/btx006.mp4

Direct injection: Procerus muscle

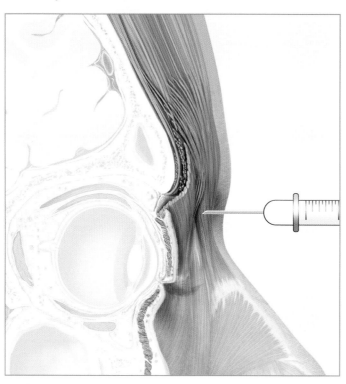

Cross-sectional anatomy, schematically demonstrating direct injection into the muscle belly of the procerus muscle.

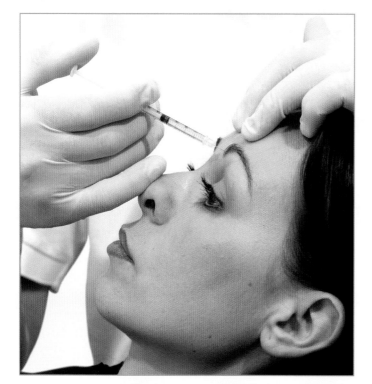

In practice, the direct injection is performed in perpendicular direction to the skin after provoked contraction of the target muscle.

4

4.7.3 Directed injection

The method known as directed injection is aimed at the site of maximum muscular tension that the patient can produce in the target muscle. This injection technique is often used for the corrugator muscle. The needle is inserted parallel to the direction of the fibers.

Video: "Directed injection technique"
http://www.kvm-tv.de/BTX/btx007.mp4

Directed injection: Corrugator muscle

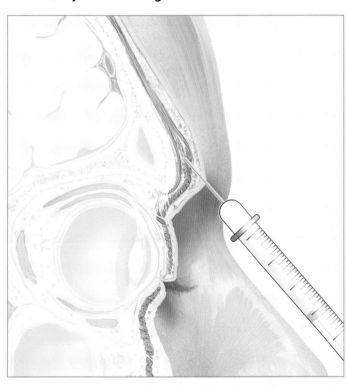

Cross-sectional anatomy, schematically showing the directed injection following the muscle fibers of the deeper-lying corrugator muscle.

4

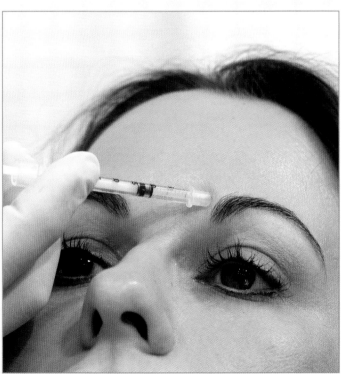

In practice, the directed injection is aimed at the side of maximal muscular tension that the patient is able to produce.

4.7.4 Two-level injection

The two-level injection is used preferentially when treating the eyebrow region. In other words the complex muscular bulk above the orbital margin consisting of the orbicularis oculi, corrugator and epicranius (frontal belly, caudal part, also referred to as Frontalis) muscles. The technique pursues the treatment goal of a natural eyebrow lift.

In the two-level injection, the active substance is injected at two levels, a deep and superficial one. The deep injection is aimed at the caudal part of the frontalis muscle. Weakening it triggers forced activity in the predominant, inferior part of the muscle acting as the only elevator of the brows. The needle is then withdrawn to a superficial level in the region of the orbicularis oculi muscle, followed by targeted intramuscular inactivation of that muscle depressing the brows in activity. Both injections will probably have further weakening effects on the contiguous corrugator muscle. Thus, use of the two-level injection achieves simultaneous stimulation of the levator (frontalis muscle) and reduction in the tone of the depressors (orbicularis oculi muscle, orbital part and corrugator muscle) leading to a maximal lifting effect.

 Video: "Two-level injection technique"
http://www.kvm-tv.de/BTX/btx008.mp4

Two-level injection: Intended effect

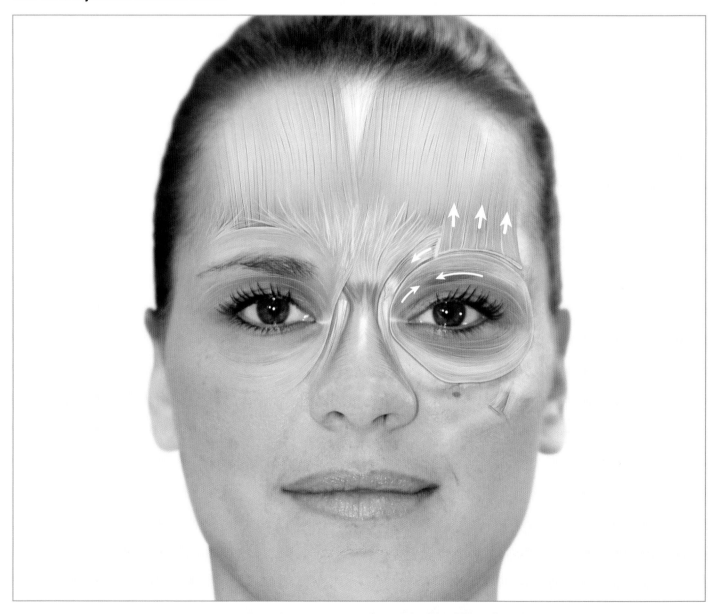

The two-level injection technique can be used along the eyebrow to achieve a natural lifting effect at two levels. By administering the toxin successively in a deeper and in a more superficial muscular layer, triggering of the elevator muscle (Frontalis) and weakening of the depressor muscles (orbicularis oculi muscle, orbital part; corrugator supercilii muscle) can be realized in one action.

Two-level injection: Performance

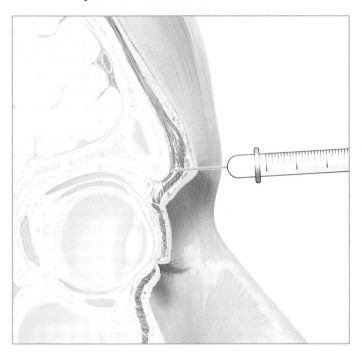

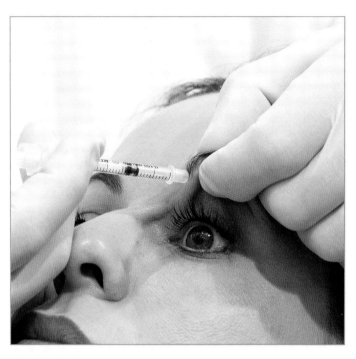

Level 1, cross-sectional anatomy: In the deep injection level, the toxin is meant to weaken central fibers of the caudal frontalis muscle. This will force the predominant, inferior part of the levator to enhanced compensatory activity.

Level 1, practice: For that purpose, the practitioner gives a deep injection first. Possible complications are prevented by isolating the muscular parts from the orbital margin with the aid of his non-injection hand.

4

Two-level injection: 2. Superficial layer

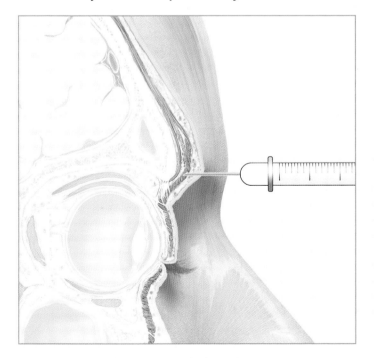

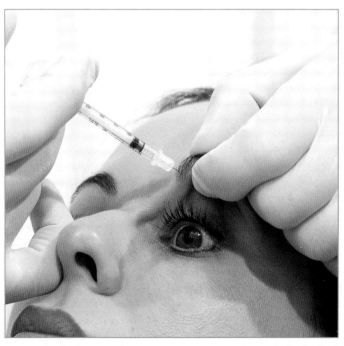

Level 2, cross-sectional anatomy: In the superficial injection level, the toxin is supposed to reach subcutaneous muscular parts. This is namely the orbital part of the orbicularis oculi muscle leading to dampened depressor activity.

Level 2, practice: The practitioner therefore withdraws the needle to a superficial level within the muscular bulk and injects another dosis targeted at the orbicularis oculi muscle.

4.7.5 Subdermal wheal technique

The so-called subdermal wheal technique provides a further option for particularly careful toxin placement. In this technique, the needle is held almost tangentially to the skin, inserting it into its uppermost layer and injecting the solution to form a subdermal wheal. This technique is used preferentially for the lower eyelid region, as the fibers of the orbicularis oculi muscle insert directly into the surface of the skin in this area. Another area where the technique is often used is the forehead. By being injected in this way, the toxin reaches the muscular target structures by diffusion.

Video: "Subdermal wheal technique"
http://www.kvm-tv.de/BTX/btx009.mp4

Subdermal wheal technique: Frontalis muscle

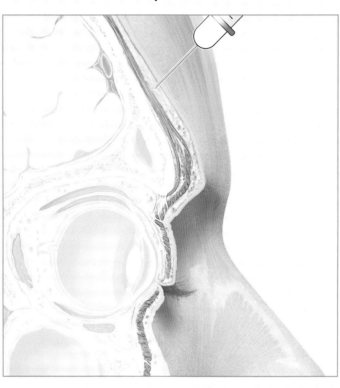

Cross-sectional anatomy, schematically demonstrating the superficial injection technique administering the substance in a subcutaneous level.

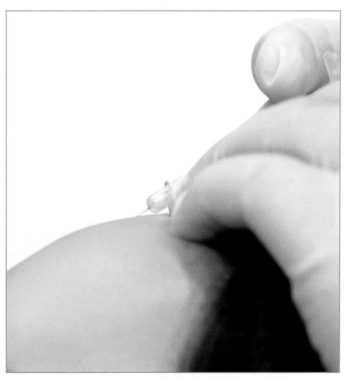

In practice, the needle is inserted nearly tangentially to the skin surface, creating a subdermal wheal by carefully injecting.

4

4.7.6 EMG-guided injection

EMG-guided injection has its advantages and disadvantages. Advantages include the more accurate localization through the acoustic signaling of the muscle activity. It may advantageous for use in very small muscles, which are difficult to distinguish such as the Levator labii superioris alaeque nasi, for relatively inexperienced injectors.

This must be weighed against disadvantages including equipment costs, the increased time input and the much thicker standard needles. The wider the needle, the more painful, unpleasant and traumatic the injection. In general terms, EMG-guided injection is rarely used in aesthetics.

4.8 Pre- and post-treatment of the face

On the day of treatment, ideally, the patient should not put on any make-up; if she does, it will need to be removed before the treatment. In very sensitive patients, an analgesic cream can be applied before giving the injections (cf. section 4.4.1, p. 29). The area being treated is disinfected before the injection with alcohol or a suitable alcohol-free antiseptic (e.g. Octenisept), which is less burning.

The injections generally cause little pain. However, minor superficial blood vessels may occasionally be punctured, causing small hematomas. The treatment areas can be cooled with cold compresses if desired.

4.9 Marking

Some therapists like to mark the treatment area or the planned injection sites before administering the injection. An ordinary cosmetic pencil is suitable for this. The advantage of marking is that the treatment can be agreed on with the patient and the proposed procedure also be explained to her. Other therapists, however, administer the injections without prior marking. In any case, marking is a useful descriptive tool that can be used to explain the planned treatment to the patient. Before the injection, the marks should be removed for hygienic reasons, although this also means that these useful mapping guides are removed.

Video: "Planning and marking of injections"
http://www.kvm-tv.de/BTX/btx010.mp4

4

Pre- and post-treatment

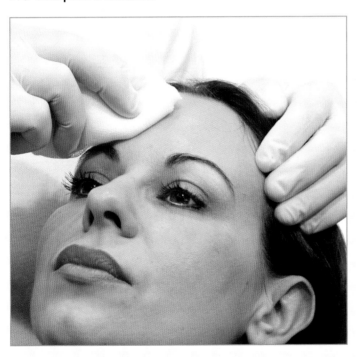

Before the treatment starts, make-up should be removed and the skin disinfected with a suitable antiseptic.

Marking

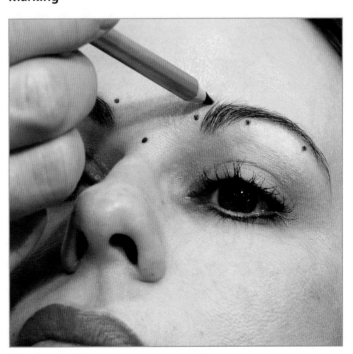

An ordinary eyebrow pencil can be used to mark the target areas.

4.10 Management of adverse treatment effects

The active substance botulinum toxin is very safe at the low doses used for dermatological indications. Side effects tend to be rare, provided that the contraindications are observed. Details of unwanted complications may be found in the description of the regional treatments (cf. Chapter 5, p. 43 ff.). The patient needs to be informed of the peculiarities of botulinum toxin treatment – such as the slow onset of action over the course of several days – during the obligatory information session. The treatment's possibilities and limitations also need to be explained beforehand. In this context, the patient should be told that botulinum toxin produces particularly good therapeutic results when used for facial expression lines. Only limited success is to be expected with age-related skin changes (actinic elastosis). Additional methods, such as augmentation with fillers and endogenous fat, or laser resurfacing, or surgery are used in these cases.

4.10.1 Unrealistic expectations

A careful evaluation of what the patient expects to gain is conducted before the treatment. By doing this, the therapist can counsel the patient regarding any unrealistic expectations.

4.10.2 Insufficient immobilization of the target muscles

Weak immobilization may be an entirely desirable result at the first treatment. The dose can be up-titrated (as it were) in one or more follow-up injections, until satisfactory immobilization is achieved.

4.10.3 Excessive immobilization of the target muscles

Excessive immobilization of the target muscles can lead to a rigid, mask-like facial expression. Thus, too much sedation of the frontal belly of the frontalis muscle makes the patient incapable of wrinkling the forehead – thus reducing the capacity for facial expression, which is desirable in a social context. Around the mouth, excessive immobilization of the orbicularis oris muscle may impair closure of the mouth, which can have a negative impact when chewing or whistling. The effect of excessive sedation can be countered by carefully feeling one's way towards the optimum dose over the course of several sessions.

4.10.4 Inadvertent immobilization of neighboring muscles

Diffusion of the toxin into neighboring muscles is one of the most unpleasant complications of botulinum toxin treatment. The periorbital area and the larynx are at risk of this. In the periorbital region, this may result in ptosis or the onset of double vision. Diffusion into the area around the larynx can lead to problems with swallowing and speech. These adverse effects can be minimized by using correct injection technique and the minimal effective dose for the treatment area.

4.10.5 Effects due to a failure to observe contraindications

The need to be aware of contraindications is an essential prerequisite of treatment with any drug, including botulinum toxin (cf. section 1.6, p. 7).

4.10.6 Local effects

Hematomas, inflammation or tenderness can develop at the injection site. According to the manufacturers' product information, there have also been isolated reports of erythema multiforme, urticaria, psoriasis-like rash, pruritus and allergic reactions.

4

5 Regional treatments

5.1 Overview of the treatment areas

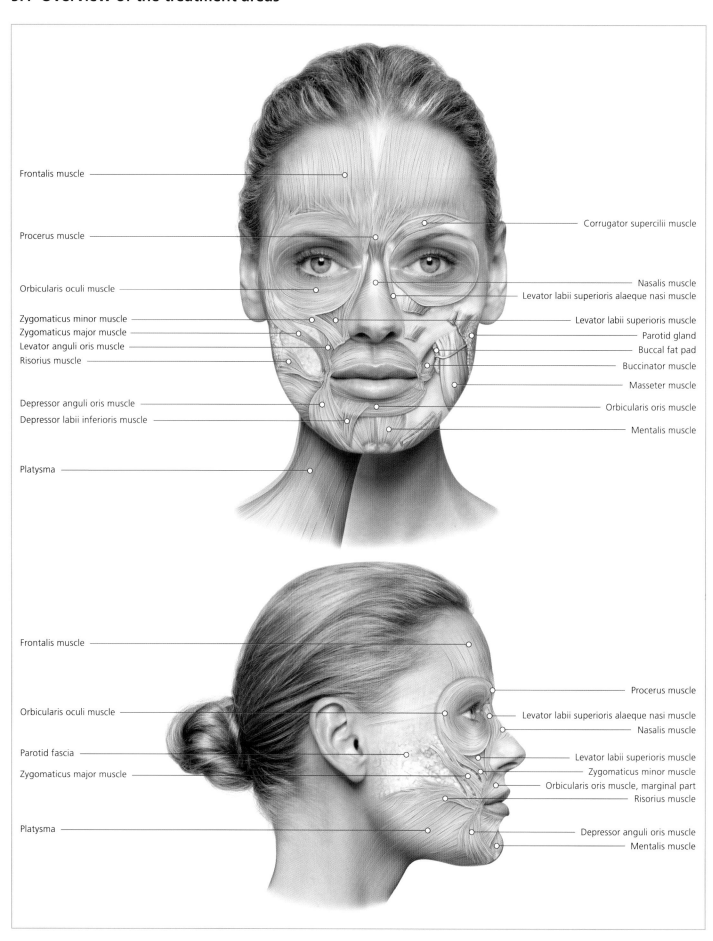

Frontalis muscle

Procerus muscle

Orbicularis oculi muscle

Zygomaticus minor muscle
Zygomaticus major muscle
Levator anguli oris muscle
Risorius muscle

Depressor anguli oris muscle
Depressor labii inferioris muscle

Platysma

Corrugator supercilii muscle

Nasalis muscle
Levator labii superioris alaeque nasi muscle

Levator labii superioris muscle
Parotid gland
Buccal fat pad
Buccinator muscle
Masseter muscle
Orbicularis oris muscle
Mentalis muscle

Frontalis muscle

Orbicularis oculi muscle

Parotid fascia

Zygomaticus major muscle

Platysma

Procerus muscle

Levator labii superioris alaeque nasi muscle
Nasalis muscle

Levator labii superioris muscle
Zygomaticus minor muscle
Orbicularis oris muscle, marginal part
Risorius muscle

Depressor anguli oris muscle
Mentalis muscle

Overview: The muscles of the face.

5

⚠ Please observe the off-label therapy warnings relating to the licensed products (cf. section 1.12, p. 8) and the relevant product inserts.

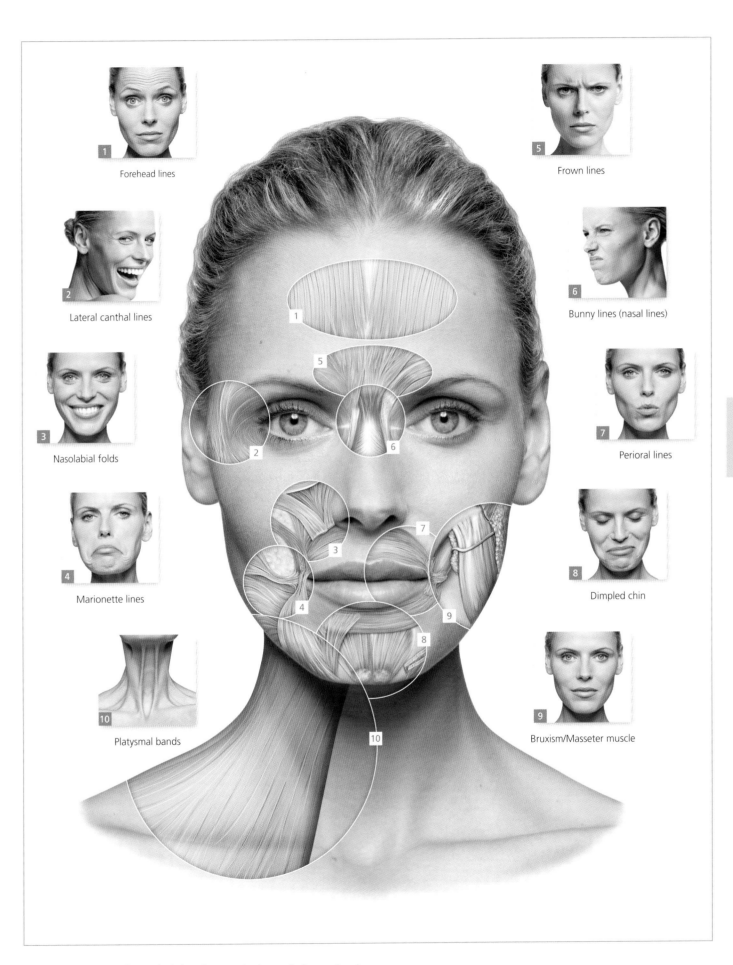

1 Forehead lines

2 Lateral canthal lines

3 Nasolabial folds

4 Marionette lines

5 Frown lines

6 Bunny lines (nasal lines)

7 Perioral lines

8 Dimpled chin

9 Bruxism/Masseter muscle

10 Platysmal bands

Overview: Indications for aesthetic botulinum toxin therapy in face and neck area.

5

5.2 Horizontal lines on the forehead | Frontalis muscle

Findings evaluation

The lines on the forehead are lines of attentiveness, which are formed when a person listens or shows interest or sympathy. They signal life experience and have positive connotations. Forehead lines have a negative effect only if they are particularly deep. These lines produced are mainly by contraction of the frontal belly of the epicranius muscle (commonly called the frontalis muscle).

5

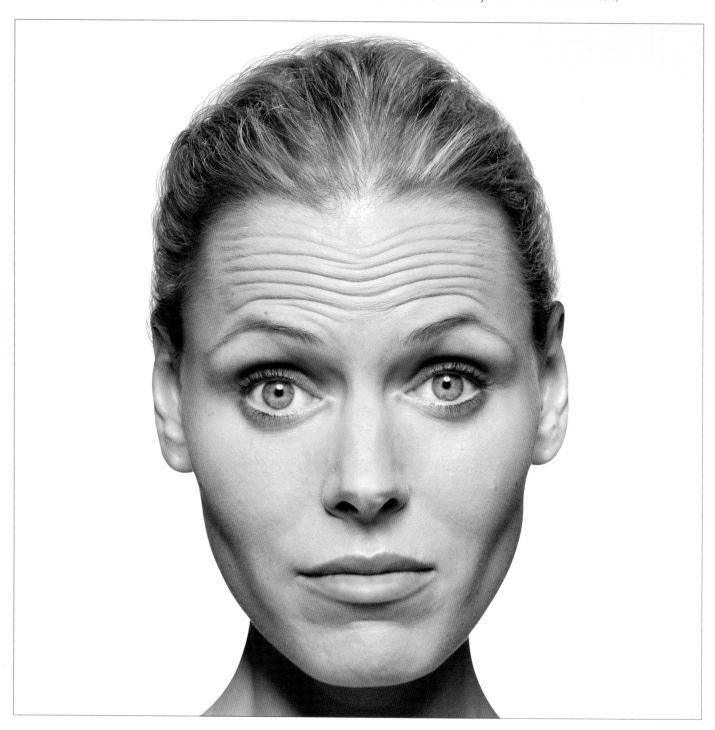

Patient selection

Very good treatment results can be expected in patients who can produce or diminish the horizontal lines by voluntary muscle contraction and relaxation. In persons with increased muscle tone, on the other hand, these lines are present both at rest and when the muscles are actively contracted. These patients are more difficult to treat, and should be warned about this during the preliminary consultation.

Assessing the indication

Horizontal forehead lines, particularly when they can be produced voluntarily and dynamically, are very responsive to treatment with botulinum toxin. The treatment effect depends on how pronounced the lines are.

⚠ Please observe the off-label therapy warnings relating to the licensed products (cf. section 1.12, p. 8) and the relevant product inserts.

Anatomy

The occipitofrontalis muscle and the usually irregular and rudimentary temporoparietalis muscle are referred to together as the epicranius muscle. The epicranius can raise the eyebrows, producing deep lines across the forehead. It is thus a significant antagonist of the orbicularis oculi muscle and opens the palpebral aperture together with the levator palpebrae superioris muscle. This takes place via the frontal part, with the help of the occipital part. By contracting, the latter secures the epicranial aponeurosis, making it the fixed point for the action of the frontal part.

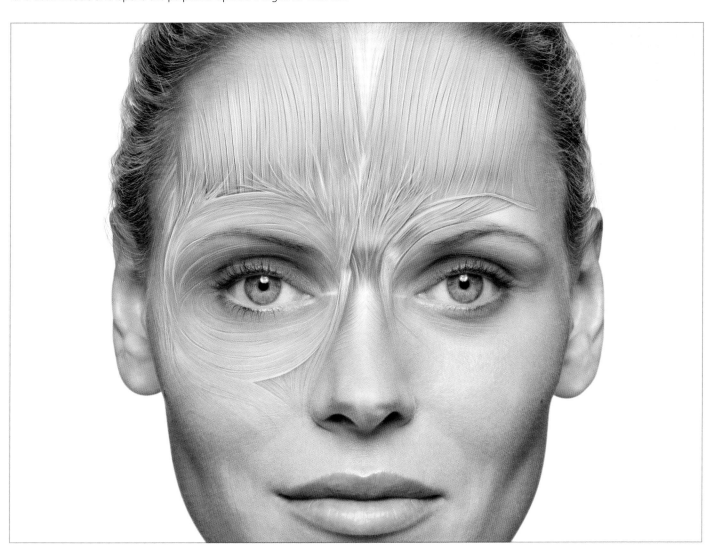

Origin
Occipitofrontalis muscle, occipital part: short, tendinous fibers from the supreme arcuate line of the occipital bone
Occipitofrontalis muscle, frontal part: the medial fibers project from the procerus muscle, the lateral fibers join with those of the corrugator supercilii and orbicularis oculi muscles
Temporoparietalis muscle: the skin of the temple, temporal fascia

Insertion
Occipitofrontalis muscle, occipital part: epicranial aponeourosis (galea aponeurotica)
Occipitofrontalis muscle, frontal part: epicranial aponeourosis, ventrally of the coronal suture
Temporoparietalis muscle: epicranial aponeourosis

Function
Raises the eyebrows

Synergists
Occipitofrontalis muscle, occipital part

Antagonists
Corrugator supercilii muscle
Procerus muscle
Depressor supercilii muscle
Orbicularis oculi muscle

Innervation
Epicranius muscle, occipital part: posterior auricular nerve from the facial nerve (cranial nerve VII)
Epicranius muscle, frontal part: temporal branches of the facial nerve (cranial nerve VII)
Temporoparietalis muscle: temporal branches of the facial nerve (cranial nerve VII)

5

Planning of treatment

The goal of the treatment is to reduce the dynamically produced lines that run across the forehead.

The frontal part of the epicranius is the only muscle that lifts the brows. Overcorrection, by overly weakening the muscle, can intensify the activity of the depressors and lead to eyebrow ptosis. This produces a cosmetically undesirable, sad or tired or angry facial expression. The effect is dose-dependent and reversible. This complication can be avoided by adjusting the dose so that adequate activation of the muscle is still possible. Furthermore, the injections need to be given a sufficient distance from the eyebrows. The brow ptosis can often be remedied by soft tissue augmentation in the eyebrow region and forehead.

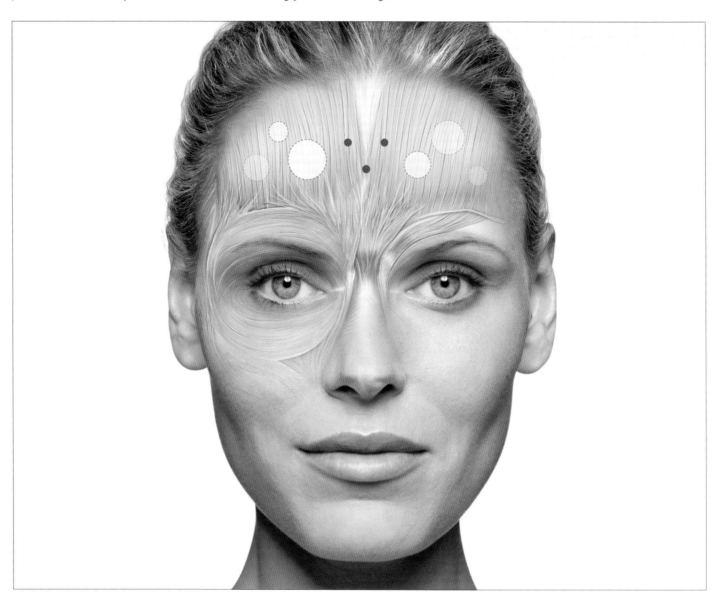

Practical tip

Overdosing and subsequent eyebrow ptosis have to be avoided when injecting into the frontalis muscle and, in particular, into its weaker lateral parts. Superficial injections at low dosages using the subdermal wheal technique are most appropriate in this respect. The authors recommend for this the use of dilutions (cf. two-third dilution, p. 32 and Chapter 5.6, p. 64 ff.) realizing maximal distribution of minimal doses, especially useful in patients at risk (i.e. pronounced wrinkling at low muscle tone).

In some cases, it is worth doing the treatment in two sessions: the glabella is treated first and the result of this awaited, as the procerus muscle may be involved in forming the lines across the forehead.

After 14 days to 4 weeks, the forehead lines can then be treated more predictably. Advanced injectors typically treat these areas at the same time.

Treatment regimen

In the medial region, deeper injections (●) administered in a V-shape into the predicted muscular region.

In the lateral region, superficial injections (◌) preferably by making use of the two-third dilution.

Caution: The lower part of the frontalis muscle (up to a distance of approx. 2 cm from the orbital margin) should better not be treated in order to prevent possible eyebrow ptosis.

⚠ Please observe the off-label therapy warnings relating to the licensed products (cf. section 1.12, p. 8) and the relevant product inserts.

Treatment

Injection

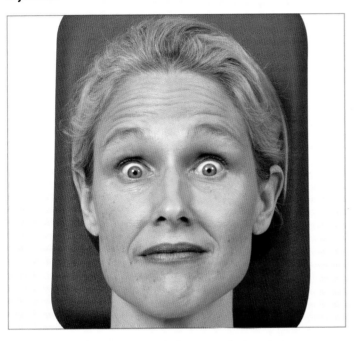

Activation
The practitioner instructs the patient to contract the muscle actively: "Raise your eyebrows and wrinkle your forehead."

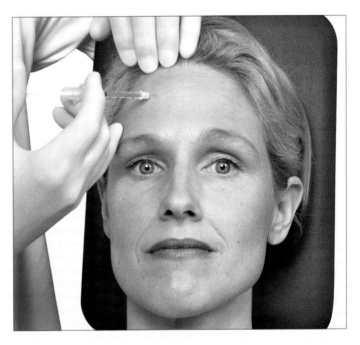

Injection technique
Direct injection with vertical insertion of the needle in the medial region. Subdermal wheal technique with tangential insertion in the lateral region.

Products and doses

Injection site	Product	Units/point	Ml solution/point
Medial frontalis muscle (in V-shape)	Xeomin	2	0.05
	Botox	2	0.05
	Dysport	5	0.025
Lateral frontalis muscle	Xeomin	0.5	0.0125 / 0.0375*
	Botox	0.5	0.0125 / 0.0375*
	Dysport	1.25	0.00625 / 0.0125**

Table 5.1 The authors' consensus dose recommendations for the treatment of horizontal front lines. * Two-third dilution ** One-half dilution. The same data apply for products with identical substance preparations. Higher doses may be needed in patients with a very high forehead. A second treatment line may need to be placed above the first if this is the case.

Correction factor

Man with active expressions: Factor 2
Age / inactive facial expressions: Factor 0.5.

Combined treatment options

It may be a good idea to supplement the treatment with superficial augmentation of residual lines or with supportive skin regeneration therapy by percutaneous collagen induction, alias Medical Needling.

Caution

There is considerable variability in the anatomy of the forehead as well as the strength of the forehead musculature, which means there is always a risk of an overtreatment and resultant eyebrow ptosis. It is essential for the injector to try to avoid this.

Complications / Managing complications

Since the frontal part of the epicranius is the only muscle that lifts the brows, an individual overtreatment leads to eyebrow ptosis. This effect is dose-dependent and reversible. The risk can be reduced by administering lower doses and considering the option of follow-up injections after 10 to 14 days. If necessary, the ptosis may be remedied by soft tissue augmentation in the eyebrow region and forehead.

If the central parts of the frontalis muscle are treated, its lateral parts may allow a certain amount of contraction in the outer regions, leading to lateral raising of the eyebrows ("Spock effect" cf. section 5.4, p. 54 ff.). This brow elevation is treated with a small dose of BTX-A injected into the lateral parts of the frontalis muscle. When performing this correction, care must be taken to inject a sufficient distance above the bony orbital margin to avoid producing eyebrow ptosis.

The lower 2 cm are often left alone when treating the frontalis muscle. Its residual activity enhances arching of the brows. Small, comma-shaped lines may form above the brows. These fine lines can be satisfactorily treated with added filler augmentation.

Video: "Treatment of horizontal forehead lines"
http://www.kvm-tv.de/BTX/btx011.mp4

5

5.3 Glabella (frown lines) | Procerus, corrugator supercilii, depressor supercilii muscles

Findings evaluation

The forehead may be said to be the "mirror of the soul," since it clearly reflects a person's mood. The frown lines are the most prominent and most telling components of human facial expression. Consequently, pronounced lines in the glabellar region give off a negative signal – regardless of the individual's actual mood, which may be positive even if frown lines are present. Relatives, friends or work colleagues will greet frown lines with comments like, "Don't look so angry!"

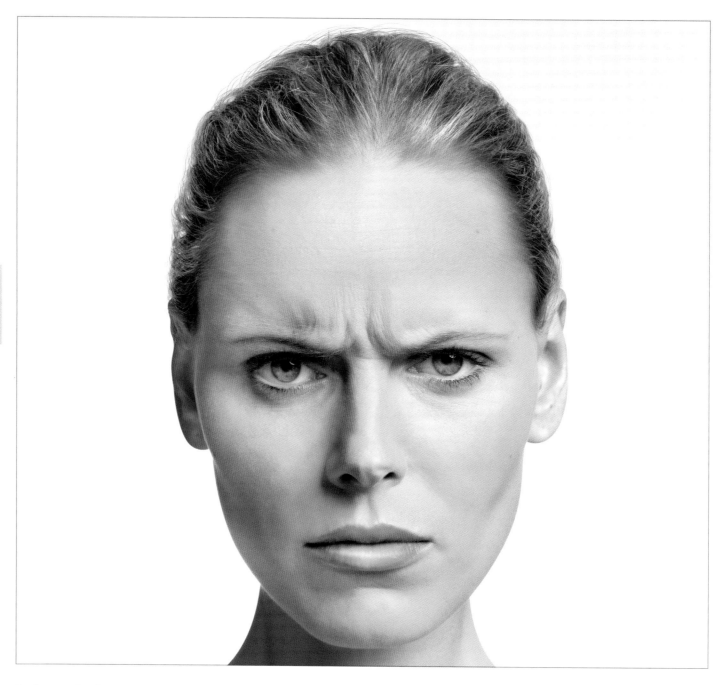

Patient selection

Very good results are to be expected in patients who can manage to produce frown lines dynamically, i.e. voluntarily.
It is also necessary to consider gender-specific differences between men and women. In men, the muscles involved are more powerful and usually need a higher dose.

Assessing the indication

Treatment of frown lines is one of the primary indications of botulinum toxin treatment. It is the only area currently approved by the FDA for cosmetic treatment with botulinum toxin. All other areas are considered sites for off-label injection.
The patient should be told that a more long-term treatment concept may lead to more successful outcomes, and that sometimes the most favorable option is to approach the desired result with smaller doses over the course of several sessions.

⚠ Please observe the off-label therapy warnings relating to the licensed products (cf. section 1.12, p. 8) and the relevant product inserts.

Anatomy

Frown lines are produced mainly by the interaction of three different muscles:

1. Procerus
2. Corrugator supercilii and
3. Depressor supercilii (orbital part of the Orbicularis oculi).

The procerus muscle, together with the corrugator supercilii muscle, pulls the skin of the medial side of the eyebrows down towards the root of the nose, thus producing deep transverse lines above it.

The corrugator supercilii muscle, together with the depressor supercilii muscle (another name for the orbital part of the orbicularis oculi muscle), draws the medial sides of the eyebrows towards the middle and downwards, thus producing vertical lines between them and over the root of the nose.

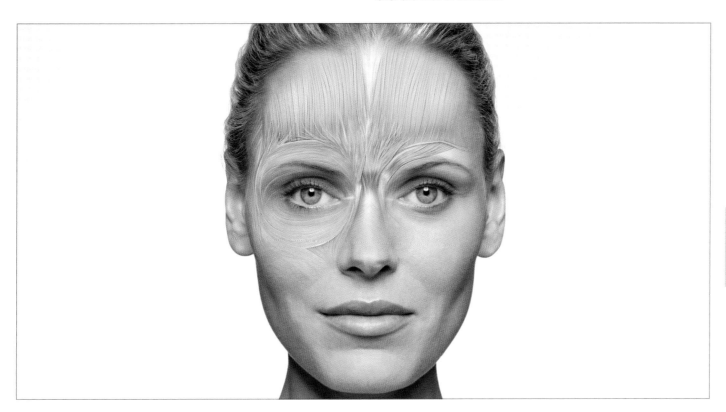

5

Procerus muscle					
Origin	**Insertion**	**Function**	**Synergists**	**Antagonists**	**Innervation**
Lower part of the nasal bone; upper part of the nasal cartilage	Skin of the forehead, between the eyebrows	Pulls the skin of the medial side of the eyebrows down towards the root of the nose	Depressor supercilii muscle Corrugator supercilii muscle Orbicularis oculi muscle	Epicranius muscle, frontal part	Temporal and zygomatic branches of the facial nerve (cranial nerve VII)
Corrugator supercilii muscle					
Nasal part of the frontal bone	Epicranial aponeurosis; skin above the middle section of the eyebrows	Draws the medial sides of the eyebrows towards the middle and downwards	Depressor supercilii muscle Orbicularis oculi muscle Procerus muscle	Epicranius muscle, frontal part	Temporal branches of the facial nerve (cranial nerve VII)
Depressor supercilii muscle (orbicularis oculi muscle, orbital part)					
Medial orbital margin close to the lacrimal bone, medial palpebral ligament	Lies in front of the corrugator supercilii muscle and radiates from it medially and into the skin of the forehead	Draws the medial sides of the eyebrows towards the meddle and downwards	Corrugator supercilii muscle Orbicularis oculi muscle Procerus muscle	Epicranius muscle, frontal part	Temporal and zygomatic branches of the facial nerve (cranial nerve VII)

Table 5.2 Some authors do not regard the depressor supercilii as a muscle in its own right, but as part of the orbicularis oculi muscle.

Planning of treatment

The goal of the treatment is to smooth out the vertical and horizontal lines in the glabellar region by partial or complete deactivation of the appropriate muscles, taking into consideration the patient's individual wishes. In this context, it will be necessary to evaluate to what extent any residual function should be preserved.

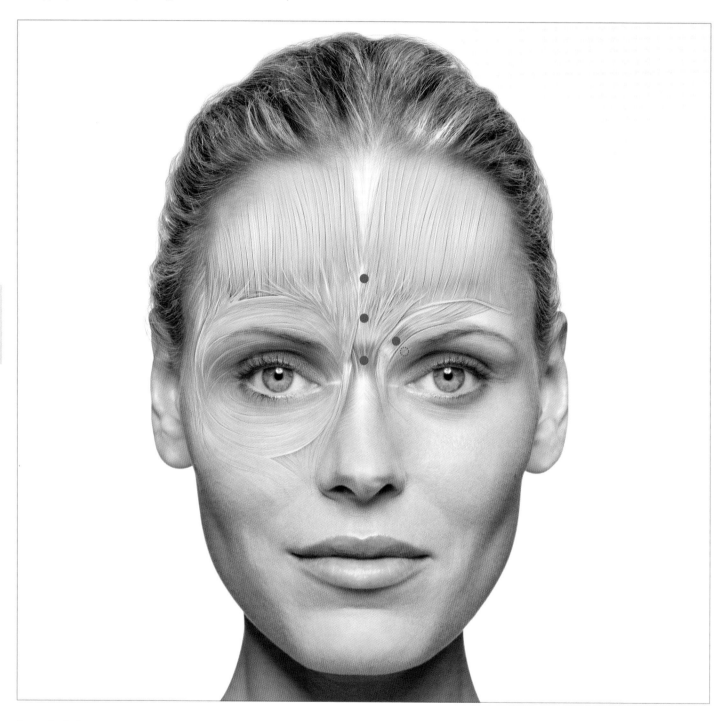

Practical tip

It is often not possible to cause any reduction in the hypertrophic muscle bellies of the corrugator muscles in a single session, especially in men. Repeated treatment of the glabellar region at 4-month intervals over a period of 1 to 2 years encourages smoothing of these lines, thus leading to a lasting effect accompanied by a reduction in the chronically hypertrophic muscle segments.

Treatment regimen

Procerus muscle: medially at the root of the nose, one to two points above that in the midline and additional injections medially and cranially into the central parts of the muscle
Corrugator supercilii muscle: one injection medially, directed along the fibers (other lateral injection points can also be considered)
Orbicularis oculi muscle, orbital part: one superficial injection (further injections along the eyebrow may be attached since a brow lift is often wished at the same time).

⚠ Please observe the off-label therapy warnings relating to the licensed products (cf. section 1.12, p. 8) and the relevant product inserts.

Treatment

Injection

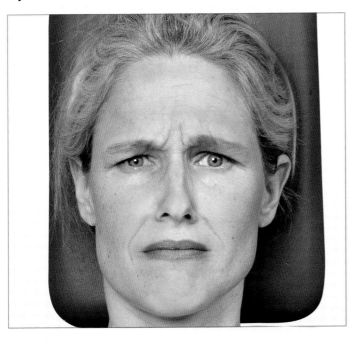

Activation
The practitioner instructs the patient to contract the muscle actively: "Pull your eyebrows together towards the nose and down," or "Frown."

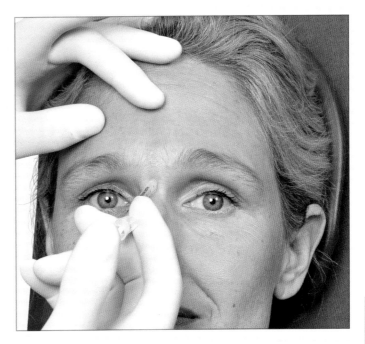

Injection technique
Procerus muscle: direct injection with vertical needle insertion
Corrugator supercilii muscle: directed injection into the center of maximum activity
Orbicularis oculi muscle, orbital part: intradermal wheal technique with tangential insertion.

Products and doses

Injection site	Product	Units/point	Ml solution/point
Procerus	Xeomin	2	0.05
	Botox	2	0.05
	Dysport	5	0.025
Corrugator supercilii	Xeomin	2–4	0.05–0.1
	Botox	2–4	0.05–0.1
	Dysport	5–10	0.025–0.05
Orbicularis oculi (orbital part)	Xeomin	1	0.025 / 0.075*
	Botox	1	0.025 / 0.075*
	Dysport	2.5	0.0125 / 0.025**

Table 5.3 The authors' consensus dose recommendations for the treatment of glabellar (frown) lines. * Two-third dilution ** One-half dilution. The same data apply for products with identical substance preparations.

Correction factor

Man with active expressions: Factor 2
Age / inactive expressions: Factor 0.5.

Combined treatment options

Soft tissue augmentation with fillers is a possible supplementary treatment option, especially for deeper lines or in older patients. A measure that can always be considered as a possible adjuvant is natural skin regeneration therapy by percutaneous collagen induction ("Medical Needling").

Complications / Managing complications

Ptosis, sometimes asymmetric, can occur after uncareful injection into the orbicularis oculi muscle due to unwanted diffusion of the toxin behind the orbital septum (cf. section 4.7.1, p. 33 ff.). If this happens, limited stimulation of the Mueller's muscle can be produced by local administration of a sympathomimetic agent such as phenylephrine (e.g. Vasocon eye drops).

Renewed intensification of the activity of the corrugator muscles may occur after 3 to 4 months, producing frown lines. In this case, follow-up injections should be given in the lateral parts of the corrugator supercilii muscle on each side.

Even if sufficient relaxation of the relevant muscles has been achieved, some individuals can produce frown lines voluntarily by recruiting the medial parts of the orbicularis oculi muscle. If this is the case, small superficial doses can be given into the palpable areas of activity of the orbicularis oculi muscle.

Slight bleeding may occur at the injection sites. This can be controlled by compression with a Q-tip (cotton bud).

Video: "Treatment of glabella lines"
http://www.kvm-tv.de/BTX/btx012.mp4

5

5.4 Eyebrows | Ideal eyebrows

The eyebrows are striking facial landmarks. Their color, position, curvature, thickness and path make a key contribution to the effect of the whole face. Low-set, hanging brows communicate a tired, weary expression in female patients. High, curved brows make the face appear fresher, younger and more awake. The eyebrows also reflect current fashion doctrine – from the thin lines of the 1920s to the perfectly arched, thicker shape of today. Gender-specific differences and preferences also need to be taken into account. Women generally prefer arched brows with a higher peak. Men tend towards straighter and more striking eyebrows. Nevertheless, the eyebrows and the individual's own facial expression need to make up a harmonious whole.

The brows can be divided into three thirds, used as reference points when describing the "ideal" eyebrow shape. However, this also requires an "ideal" eye position, in which the distance between the eyes equals the width of one eye. The first two thirds of the eyebrows rise gently from the medial to the lateral ends, after which they slope downwards slightly. The reference points can be illustrated using three imaginary lines.

5

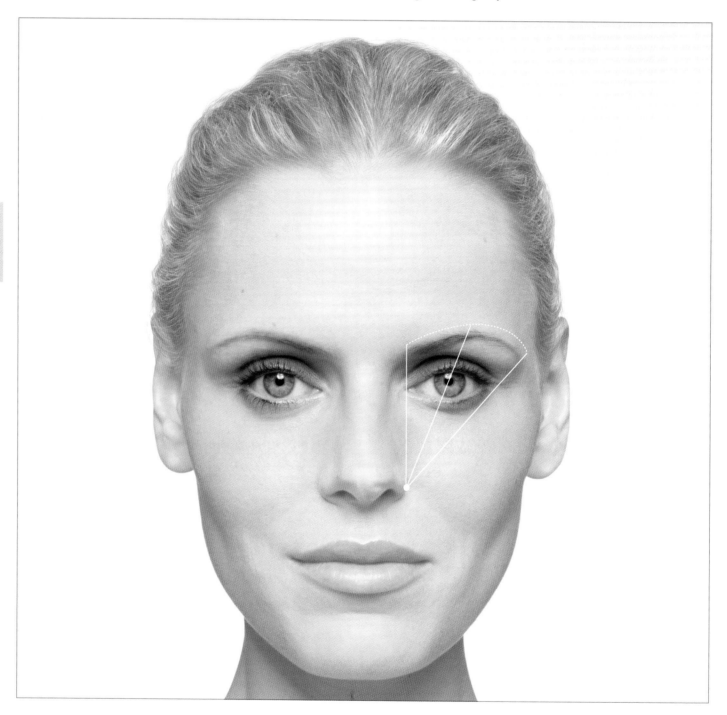

Eyebrow starting point: on the vertical line that runs upwards from the outermost point of the wing of the nose
Arch or peak: the line connecting the wing of the nose, the pupil and the brow

Eyebrow end point: the line connecting the wing of the nose, the lateral corner of the eye and the end of the brow (any brow hairs growing past this point may disrupt the overall harmony of the face).

Please observe the off-label therapy warnings relating to the licensed products (cf. section 1.12, p. 8) and the relevant product inserts.

Anatomy

The movement of the brows represents a complex interaction between several muscles. An understanding of this interaction is important if targeted interventions are to be undertaken. The following muscles are directly involved in the movement of the brows:

- frontalis muscle
- orbicularis oculi muscle
- corrugator supercilii muscle
- depressor supercilii muscle
- procerus muscle.

The frontal part of the epicranius (frontalis muscle) is the only muscle that can raise the brows actively. The remaining muscles act as antagonists to this action. The corrugator supercilii and the depressor supercilii muscles work together to pull the medial sides of the eyebrows towards the middle and downwards. The procerus, together with the corrugator supercilii, pulls the skin on the medial side of the eyebrows towards the root of the nose, reducing the medial distance between the eyebrows.

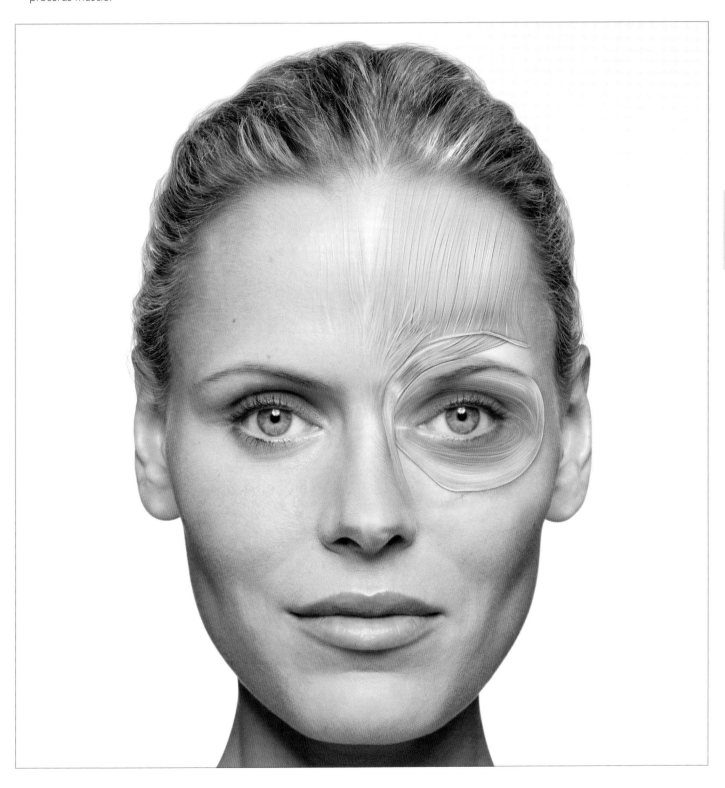

5

Chemical brow lift

Changes to the eyebrows during the natural ageing process

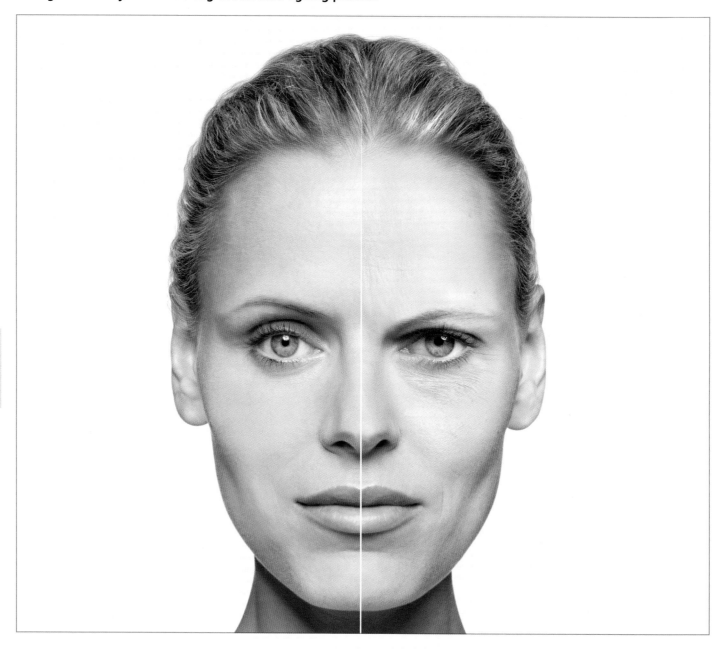

Split-face illustration to visualize the physiological ageing processes in the eyebrow region: youthful, curved eyebrow form in common with an appealing and awaked look (right side of the face) versus lowered eyebrow with drooping lid and tired look at advanced aging (left side).

Findings evaluation

One of the phenomena that occurs as part of the normal aging processes in the forehead is sinking of the brows, particularly in the lateral segment. Aging is also associated with a loss of eyebrow arching and height.

Patient selection

Individuals who can raise their eyebrows voluntarily and actively to a relevant extent benefit most from the treatment. A good assessment of the dynamics of this process can be made during the preliminary consultation, simply by observing the patient. Patients should be warned that an asymmetry in eyebrow height may occur after the treatment. This is treated with a follow-up injection. Important: in case of asymmetry, in general it is best to attempt to raise the lower brow to match the higher one.

Assessing the indication

The administration of botulinum toxin helps produce an alert, attentive, interested and anxiety-free facial expression. It could either represent a non-invasive alternative to a surgical brow lift or be used to postpone a scheduled brow lift to a later date.

⚠ Please observe the off-label therapy warnings relating to the licensed products (cf. section 1.12, p. 8) and the relevant product inserts.

Planning of treatment

The treatment goal is to lift the brows. To do this, the depressor function of the orbicularis oculi (orbicular part) and of the corrugator supercilii and procerus muscles needs to be reduced, while the elevating activity of the frontalis muscle should be triggered. It should be said that the procerus and corrugator supercilii muscles only have a supportive effect, in that they move the brows in the medial direction and slightly downwards.

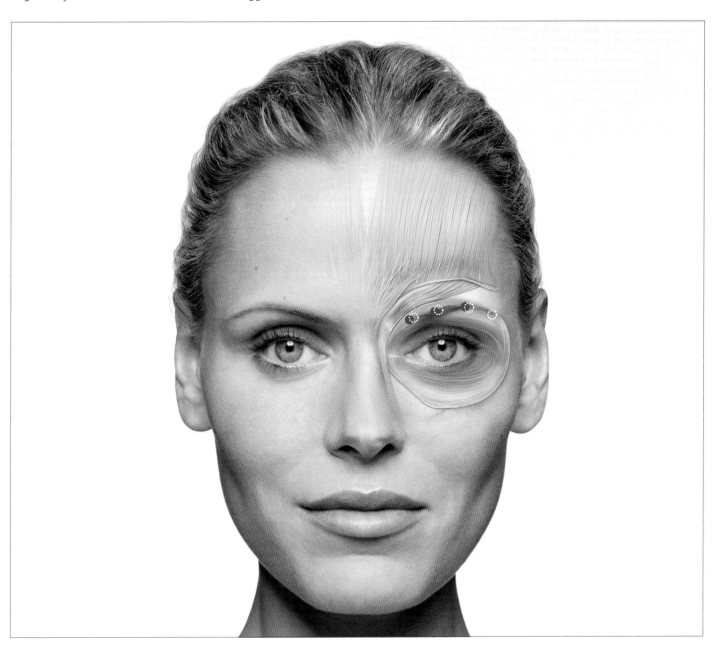

5

Practical tip

The anatomical and functional variability of the brow and forehead region has to be considered in individual planning of treatment, so the number of injection sites and doses may differ, not only between patients but also between the left and the right eyebrow. The biggest lifting effect can be achieved by injecting the substance at two depth levels, reaching a dose-dependent weakening of the deeper muscle parts (corrugator and frontalis muscle) and of the subcutaneous orbicularis oculi muscle at the same time. With the aid of the non-injection hand, the practitioner should segregate the muscular parts during injection at highest distance from the orbital margin to prevent ptosis.

Treatment regimen

The active substance is mostly administered into four sites along the eyebrow above the bony orbital margin. At the median sites, injections are usually given at two depths into the muscle layer, either by applying in an upper and a lower row or by making use of the two-level technique. The fibers of the orbicularis muscle are treated by superficial injection (inferior injection points), whereas deeper injections (superior injection points) are supposed to reach the caudal parts of the frontalis and fibers of the corrugator supercilii muscle. At the lateral site, only superficial injections are given.

Treatment

Injection

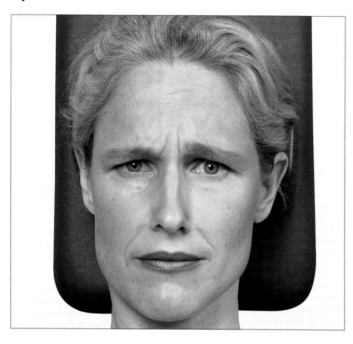

Activation
The practitioner instructs the patient to contract the muscle actively: "Pull your eyebrows down and give me a really angry look."

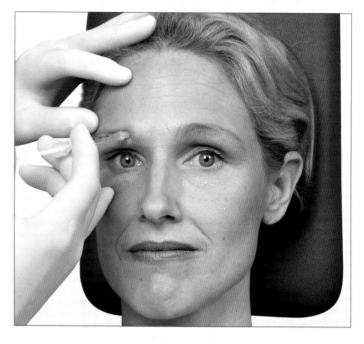

Injection technique
The injections are given at two depths, i.e. using the two-level technique (cf. section 4.7.3, p. 37) or applying in two rows. The intramuscular injection – as shown here – is given further down, inserting the needle perpendicularly to the skin. The needle should not touch the periosteum. Further superficial injection are given to damp the orbicularis oculi muscle.

Products and doses

Injection site	Product	Units/point	Ml solution/point
Medial eyebrow, deep level	**Xeomin**	2	0.05
	Botox	2	0.05
	Dysport	5	0.025
Medial eyebrow, superficial level	**Xeomin**	1	0.025 / 0.075*
	Botox	1	0.025 / 0.075*
	Dysport	2.5	0.0125 / 0.025**
Lateral eyebrow, superficial level	**Xeomin**	1	0.025 / 0.075*
	Botox	1	0.025 / 0.075*
	Dysport	2.5	0.0125 / 0.025**

Table 5.4 The authors' consensus dose recommendations for the treatment of glabellar (frown) lines. * Two-third dilution ** One-half dilution. The same data apply for products with identical substance preparations.

Correction factor

Man with active expressions: Factor 2
Age / inactive expressions: Factor 0.5.

Combined treatment options

After 1 to 2 weeks, volume fillers can be injected under the eyebrows, with the aim of lifting the brows and emphasizing their ventral region. The augmentation treatment is often carried out in multiple sessions due to the deep injection below the orbicularis oculi muscle and to avoid creating a heavy brow. Further, percutaneous collagen induction therapy (alias Medical Needling) is also able to achieve significant lifting effects and may be considered as a good adjuvant measure to achieve lasting improvement.

Complications / Managing complications

Care must be taken in two different respects: firstly, unwanted diffusion of the toxin behind the orbital septum can cause ptosis what usually should be avoided beforehand by protecting the epicranial aponeurosis from possible damage with careful injections in maximal distance to the bony boundary (cf. section 4.7.1, p. 33 ff.). If ptosis happens, limited stimulation of the tarsalis superior muscle can be produced by local administration of a sympathomimetic agent such as phenylephrine (e.g. Vasocon eye drops).
Furthermore, weakening of the lateral depressor (orbicularis oculi muscle) and medial elevator activity (frontalis muscle) quickly result in hyperactivity of the lateral muscle parts of the elevating frontalis muscle causing the so-called "Spock effect."

Video: "Chemical brow lift"
http://www.kvm-tv.de/BTX/btx013.mp4

⚠ Please observe the off-label therapy warnings relating to the licensed products (cf. section 1.12, p. 8) and the relevant product inserts.

Spock effect (Mephisto look)

Findings evaluation

The Spock effect (also knows as the Mephisto look) is not a typical indication, but in fact a side effect which can occur following forehead treatment and eyebrow correction. The Spock effect, i.e. the lateral raising of the eyebrow, results from weakening of the medial side of the frontalis muscle. This can produce compensatory hyperactivity of the lateral side of the muscle, raising the lateral segment of the eyebrow.

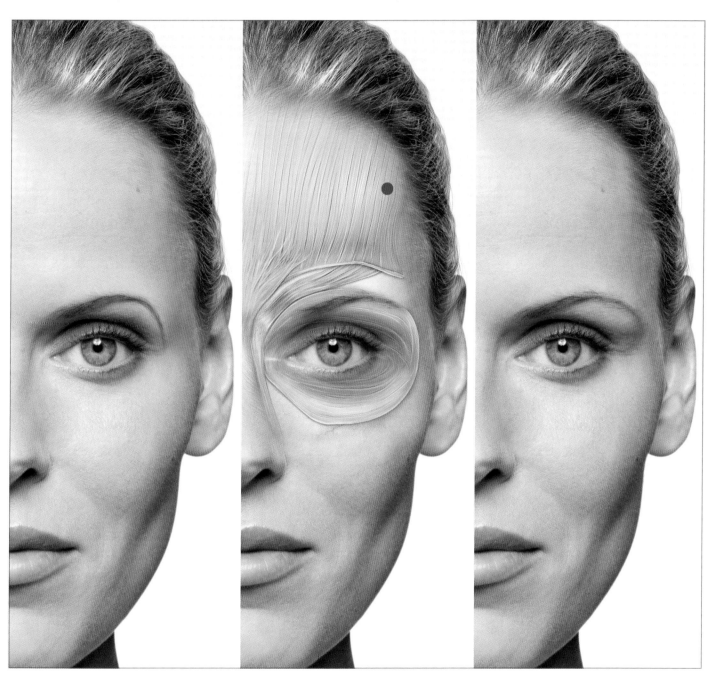

Treatment regimen

One low-dosed injection into the lateral side of the frontalis muscle at a sufficient distance (approx. 2 cm) from the eyebrow.

Products and doses

Injection site	Product	Units/point	Ml solution/point
Medial eyebrow, deep level	Xeomin	1	0.025 / 0.075*
	Botox	1	0.025 / 0.075*
	Dysport	2.5	0.0125 / 0.025**

Table 5.5 * Two-third dilution ** One-half dilution.

Correction factor

Man with active expressions:	Factor 2
Age / inactive expressions:	Factor 0.5

 Complications / Managing complications

An injection too close to the eyebrow can cause general brow ptosis. An excessive dose may cause overcorrection, leading to the lateral part of the eyebrow to hang too low.

5.5 Lateral canthal lines | Orbicularis oculi muscle

Findings evaluation

The area around the eyes is one of the most interesting parts of the face. People communicate with their eyes, allowing us to interpret their reactions and feelings. In essence, laughter lines radiate positivity. The lines are formed when the smooth, radial course of the in-dividual lines becomes broken up. Skin thickness and the age-related changes in its elasticity also affect the depth and length of these lines. People with thicker skin have deeper lines, while people with thinner skin exhibit finer and more superficial wrinkling.

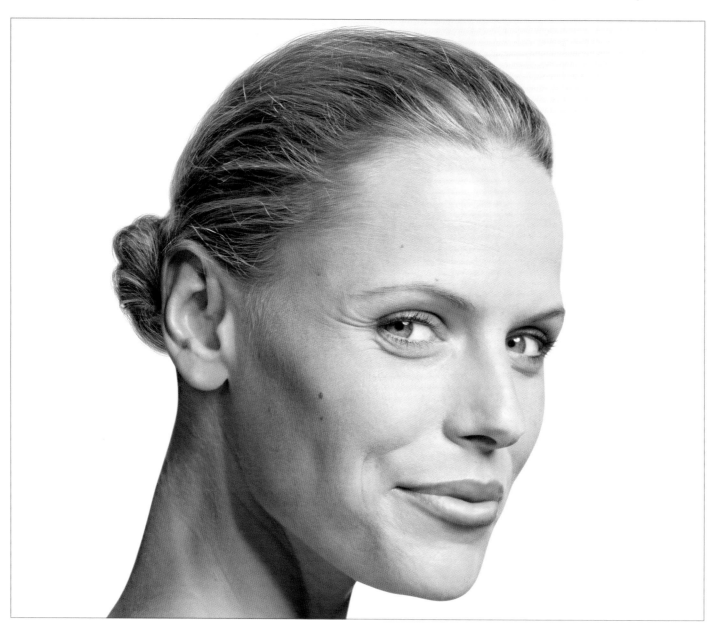

Patient selection

It will be necessary to distinguish between static and dynamic lines. The chances of success are best in individuals who can produce the lines actively (e.g. when laughing or squinting). Changes due to advanced actinic elastosis with an increase in static lines and irregular pigmentation, occurring predominantly in older people with a fair complexion, respond less well to treatment with botulinum toxin alone.

Any unrealistic expectations held by the patients need to be put into perspective before the treatment, to avoid disappointment. E.g. while it may well be possible to minimize the dynamic lines, the sta-tic lines could become more pronounced and more noticeable, a situation the patient will regard as a "treatment failure."

Men normally ask for a partial reduction of the orbital lines and will be happy if that is achieved. In contrast, women often want complete reduction of the lateral eye lines.

Assessing the indication

Botulinum toxin is well suited for the treatment of periorbital lines, particularly if they can be produced voluntarily by the patient.

⚠ Please observe the off-label therapy warnings relating to the licensed products (cf. section 1.12, p. 8) and the relevant product inserts.

Anatomy

The orbicularis oculi muscle, with its two parts, the palpebral and the orbital, can cause narrowing of the palpebral aperture; it thus acts as an antagonist to the levator palpebrae superioris muscle and to the tarsalis superior and tarsalis inferior muscles. When a person laughs or smiles it produces the typical laughter lines, which radiate outwards from the lateral corner of the eye. Depending on the individual extent of the muscle, these lines may run all the way into the cheek region.

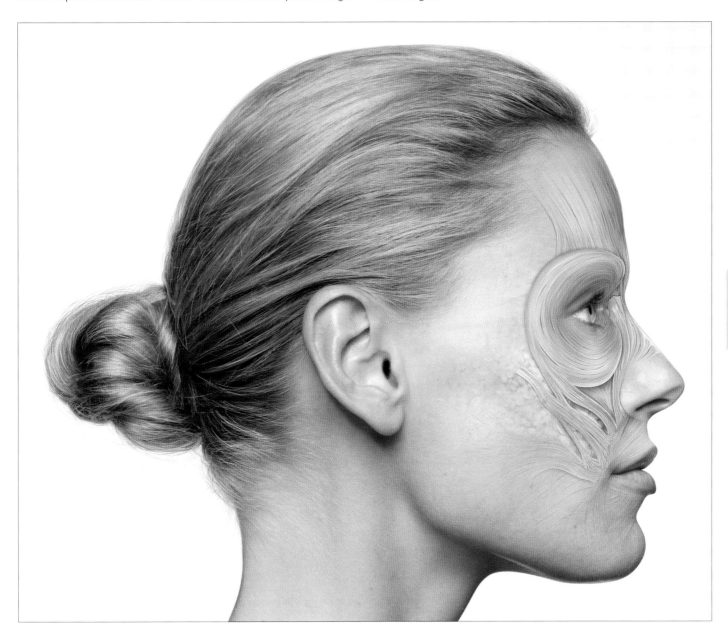

5

Origin
Medial part of the orbit (nasal part of the frontal process of the maxilla, anterior lacrimal crest and medial palpebral ligament)

Insertion
Palpebral part: skin of the upper and lower eyelids
Orbital part: fanning out broadly to attach to the skin of the orbit, the forehead and the cheeks

Function
Narrows the palpebral fissure with its palpebral and orbital parts
Antagonist of the levator palpebrae superioris muscle and the tarsalis superior and inferior muscles

Synergists
Corrugator supercilii muscle
Procerus muscle

Antagonists
Levator palpebrae superioris muscle
Tarsalis superior and inferior muscles
Epicranius muscle, frontal part

Innervation
Temporal and zygomatic branches of the facial nerve (cranial nerve VII)

Planning of treatment

The target structure is the orbital part of the orbicularis oculi muscle. The treatment goal is to reduce any voluntarily produced, dynamic lines and/or to smooth out lines which occur as a result of hypertonic muscle activity at rest.

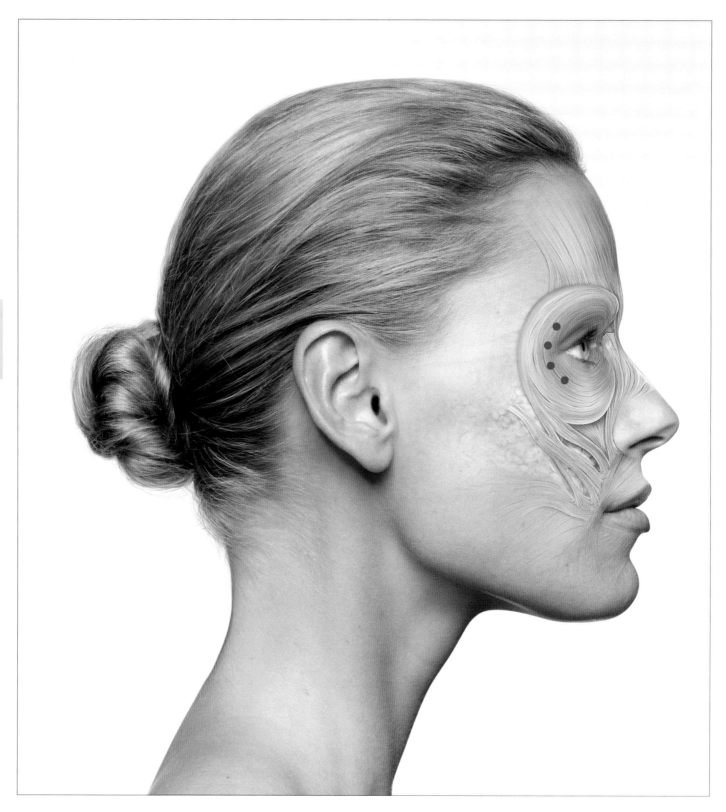

Practical tip

Some authors recommend frequent injection at intervals of 4 to 6 weeks – each time at a low dose – for lasting smoothening of the lines. However, that procedure has drawn criticism from the FDA.

Treatment regimen

Deeper, subcutaneous injections are given over the lateral bony margin of the orbit.

⚠ Please observe the off-label therapy warnings relating to the licensed products (cf. section 1.12, p. 8) and the relevant product inserts.

Treatment

Injection

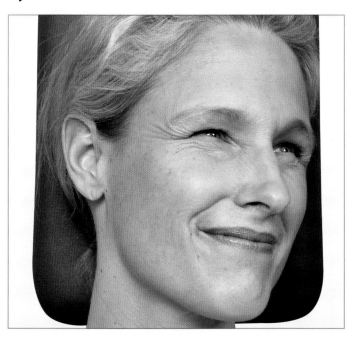

Activation
The practitioner instructs the patient to contract the muscle actively: "Give me your most radiant smile!"

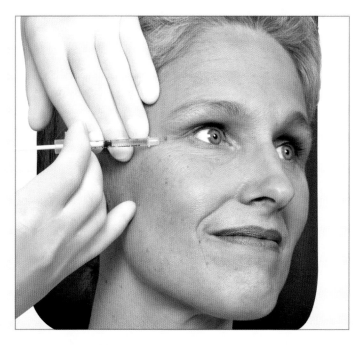

Injection technique
Administer slightly deeper, subcutaneous injections over the bony orbital margin, inserting the needle vertically.

Products and doses

Injection site	Product	Units/point	MI solution/point
Lateral orbicularis oculi muscle	**Xeomin**	1	0.025
	Botox	1	0.025
	Dysport	2.5	0.0125

Table 5.6 The authors' consensus dose recommendations for the treatment of lateral canthal lines. The same data apply for products with identical substance preparations.

Correction factor
Man with active expressions: Factor 2
Age / inactive expressions: Factor 0.5.

Combined treatment options
The treatment may be combined with augmentation methods (fillers, endogenous fat), especially if pronounced static lines are present. Various resurfacing techniques can also be very useful in this area if the patient can tolerate downtime for recovery. A further option to supplement the result is via percutaneous collagen induction, which is a riskless and nearly downtime-free skin regeneration method notably useful in the sensitive area around the eyes.

Caution
If combining the treatment with laser resurfacing or deep peels, the resultant inflammatory stimulus increases the permeability of the tissues and the diffusion potential of the botulinum toxin. The risk of complications may increase, while the treatment outcome becomes less predictable.

Complications / Managing complications

Injecting too deep into the lateral region of the orbicularis oculi (orbital part) can lead to inactivation of the zygomatic muscles. This in turn leads to reduced contractility of the cheek muscles, altering the smile.
Slight bleeding may occur at the injection sites. This can be controlled by compression with a Q-tip (cotton bud).
In rare cases, the toxin may diffuse into the lateral eye muscles, leading to double vision.
Caution is needed in patients with prominent tear troughs, as these bags under the eyes can be enhanced by further reduction in the tone of the orbicularis oculi muscle, producing a pseudo-hernia.
Injections too close to the edge of the lower lid can cause it to sag, i.e. they can produce ectropion or lower lid retraction.

5

5.6 Fine skin creases on the lower eyelid | Orbicularis oculi muscle

Findings evaluation

Fine skin creases on the lower eyelid are formed when the skin's surface is puckered by the activity of the orbicular part of the orbicularis oculi, which is directly attached to the skin. This activity is triggered when blinking and when squinting into very bright light, and is seen particularly in fair-skinned, blue-eyed people with red or blond hair. Other predisposing factors include age-related loss of skin elasticity, as well as external influences such as cold, wind, and nicotine.

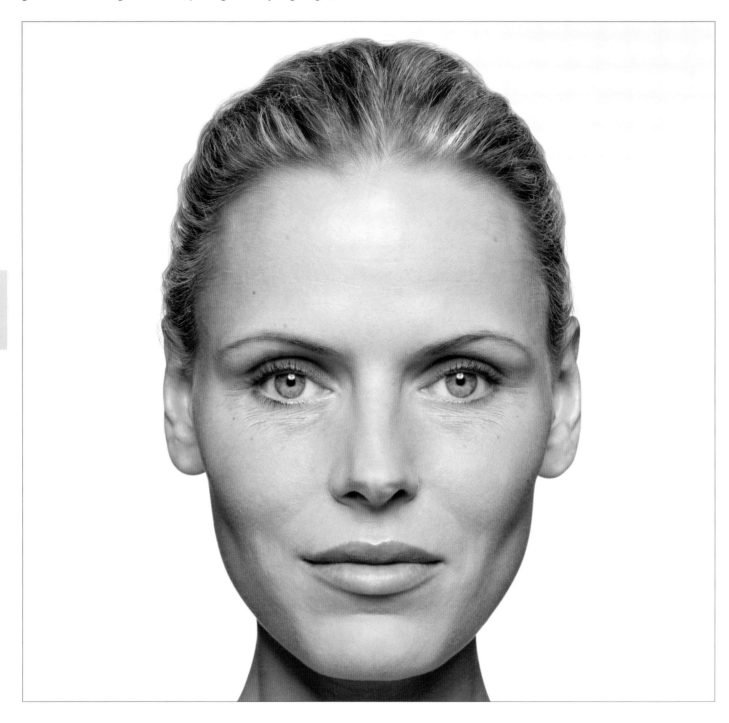

Patient selection

Younger patients whose tissues still retain their elasticity benefit most from this treatment. The elasticity of the skin below the eyes can be tested with the snap-back test (cf. section 3.3, p. 24 f.).
Loss of tone of the orbicularis oculi muscle can cause bags (pseudohernias) referred to as tear troughs to appear below the eyes. This situation can be made even worse by using botulinum toxin A, giving the patient's face a tired look. Therefore, botulinum toxin A should only be given by very experienced injectors to patients with pronounced tear troughs or prominent infraorbital fat.

Assessing the indication

Well suited for smoothing of the skin below the eyes, provided the skin retains its elasticity and subject to good patient selection.

⚠ Please observe the off-label therapy warnings relating to the licensed products (cf. section 1.12, p. 8) and the relevant product inserts.

Anatomy

The orbicularis oculi muscle, with its two parts, the palpebral and the orbital, can cause narrowing of the palpebral aperture; it thus acts as an antagonist to the levator palpebrae superioris muscle and to the tarsalis superior and inferior muscles. When a person laughs or smi-

les it produces the typical laugh lines, which radiate outwards from the lateral corner of the eye. Depending on the individual extent of the muscle, these lines may run all the way into the cheek region.

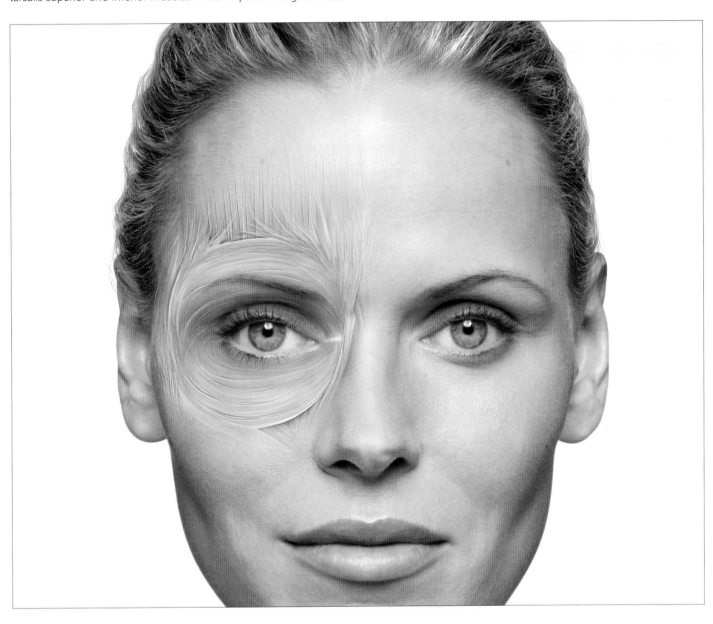

Origin
Medial part of the orbit (nasal part of the frontal process of the maxilla, anterior lacrimal crest and medial palpebral ligament)

Insertion
Palpebral part: skin of the upper and lower eyelids
Orbital part: fanning out broadly to attach to the skin of the orbit, the forehead and the cheeks

Function
Narrows the palpebral fissure with its palpebral (often further subdivided into the pretarsal and preseptal parts) and orbital parts
Antagonist of the levator palpebrae superioris muscle and the tarsalis superior and inferior muscles

Synergists
Corrugator supercilii muscle
Procerus muscle

Antagonists
Levator palpebrae superioris muscle
Tarsalis superior and inferior muscles
Epicranius muscle, frontal part

Innervation
Temporal and zygomatic branches of the facial nerve (cranial nerve VII)

5

Planning of treatment

The goal of the botulinum toxin treatment is to smooth the skin under the eyes. This is done with very small doses of the drug, which is administered by intradermal injection, allowing it to diffuse into the orbicularis muscle (orbital part).

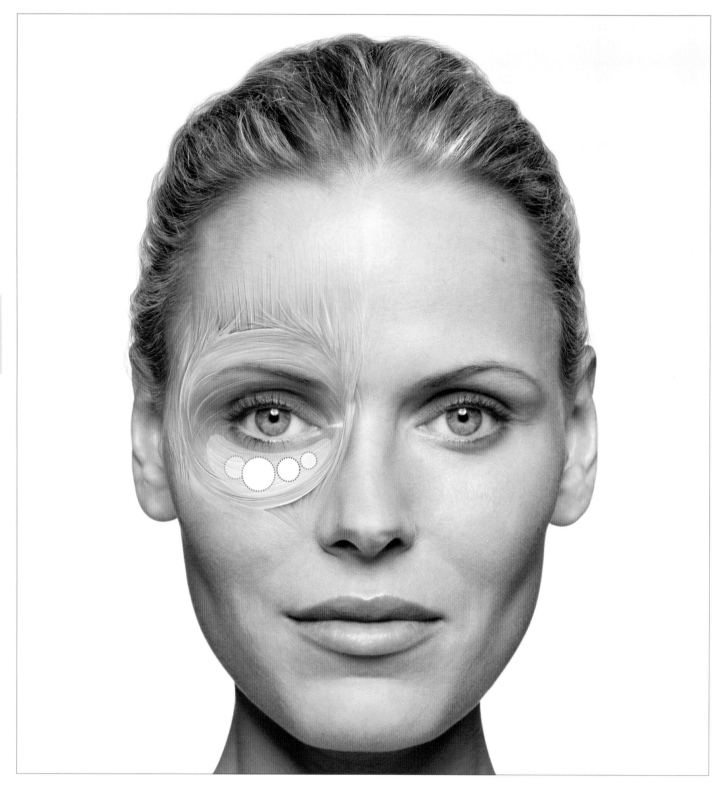

Practical tip

Fine lines on the lower eyelid are best treated with dilutions of the standard solutions (e.g. "two-third dilution" of Xeomin/Botox, one-half dilution of Dysport, cf. section 4.6, p. 32) allowing a maximal range of diffusion in the use of minimal doses.

Treatment regimen

Four strictly intradermal depots at minimal doses using dilutions of the standard solutions are administered into the infraorbital region where the fine lines are located.

⚠ Please observe the off-label therapy warnings relating to the licensed products (cf. section 1.12, p. 8) and the relevant product inserts.

Treatment

Injection

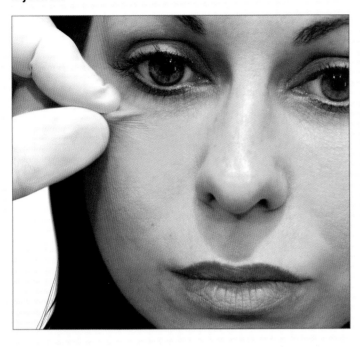

Snap-back test
The practitioner tests tissue elasticity and turgor with the snap-back test (cf. section 3.3, p. 24).

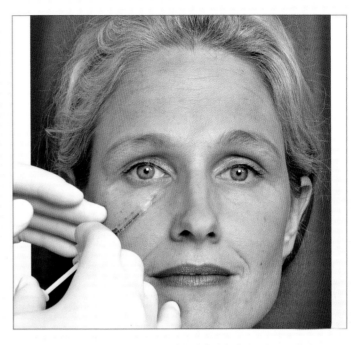

Injection technique
Four intradermal depots of minimal dose each are administered into the lower eyelid region by superficial subcutaneous injection. The needle is inserted tangentially to the skin. After the injection, the area may be massaged gently to ensure uniform distribution of the active substance. To avoid perforating smaller blood vessels, the skin can be stretched slightly before it is injected.

Products and doses

Injection site	Product	Units/point	Ml solution/point
Infraorbital region	Xeomin®	0.5	0.0375*
	Botox®	0.5	0.0375*
	Dysport®	1.25	0.0125**

Table 5.7 The authors' consensus dose recommendations for the treatment of fine lines on the lower eyelid. * Two-third dilution ** One-half dilution. The same data apply for products with identical substance preparations.

Correction factor

Man with active expressions: Factor 2
Age / inactive expressions: Factor 0.5.

Combined treatment options

Very suitable in combination with percutaneous collagen induction therapy, subsurfacing (fractional photothermolysis) or fractional laser resurfacing (e.g. Fraxel repair), provided that the injector is experienced. In these cases, the authors administer botulinum toxin before the other scheduled treatment measures.

 Complications / Managing complications

Caution is needed in patients with prominent infraorbital fat or "tear troughs," as these can be enhanced by further reduction in the tone of the orbicularis oculi muscle, which produces a pseudohernia.

Slight bleeding may occur at the injection sites. This can be controlled by compression with a Q-tip (cotton bud). Rarely, lymphedema may result due to the decreased pumping mechanism of the orbicularis oculi muscle.

Small hematomas may develop at the puncture sites; these resolve after 1 to 2 weeks.

Injections too close to the edge of the lower lid or in a weak lower lid can cause it to sag, i.e. they can produce ectropion or lid retraction.

5

5.7 Open eye (widening the palpebral aperture) | Orbicularis oculi muscle

Findings evaluation

The pretarsal part of the orbicularis oculi muscle can hypertrophy and reduce the vertical size of the palpebral aperture, particularly in persons of Asian origin. Therefore, requests for aesthetic widening of the palpebral aperture tend to come mainly from that ethnic group.

Palpebral aperture widening has therapeutic significance in individuals with idiopathic asymmetry of the eyes. The visible part of the eyeball is enlarged by means of a slight distal displacement of the lower edge of the eyelid.

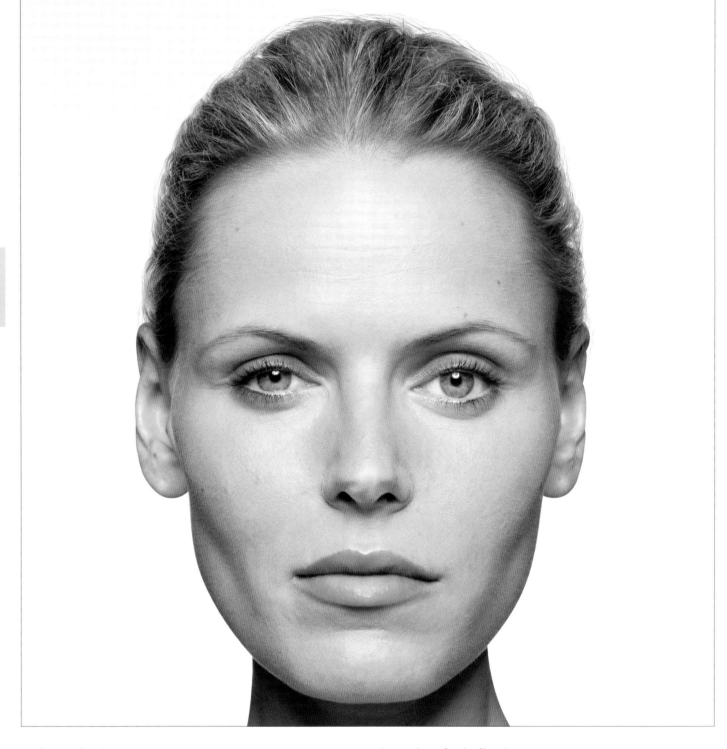

Patient selection

Younger patients whose tissues still retain their elasticity benefit most from this treatment. The elasticity of the skin below the eyes should be tested with the snap-back test (cf. section 3.3, p. 24).

Assessing the indication

Suitable only for experienced therapists; this tends to be a rare indication in European countries.

⚠ Please observe the off-label therapy warnings relating to the licensed products (cf. section 1.12, p. 8) and the relevant product inserts.

Anatomy

The orbicularis oculi muscle, with its two parts, the palpebral and the orbital, can cause narrowing of the palpebral aperture; it thus acts as an antagonist to the levator palpebrae superioris muscle and to the tarsalis superior and inferior muscles.

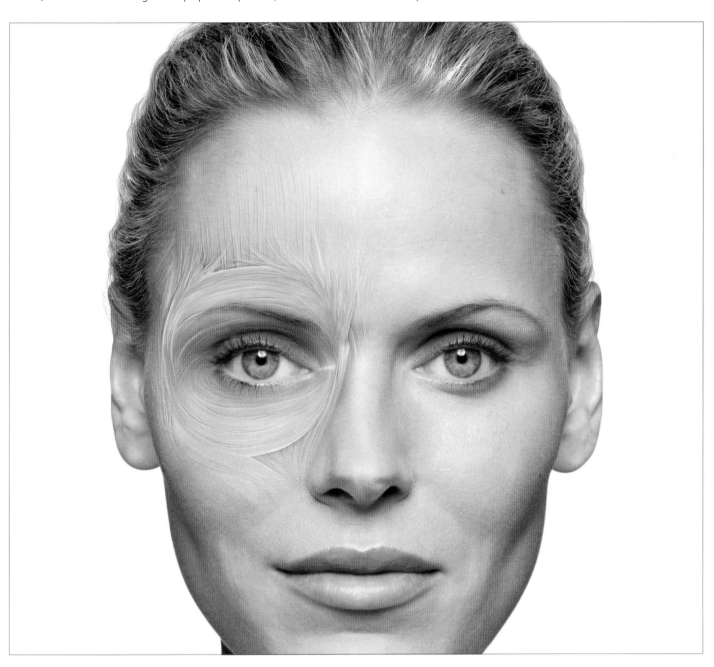

Origin
Medial part of the orbit (nasal part of the frontal process of the maxilla, anterior lacrimal crest and medial palpebral ligament)

Insertion
Palpebral part: skin of the upper and lower eyelids
Orbital part: fanning out broadly to attach to the skin of the orbit, the forehead and the cheeks

Function
Narrowing of the palpebral fissure by the pleural and orbital parts
Antagonist of the levator palpebrae superioris muscle and the tarsalis superior and inferior muscles

Synergists
Corrugator supercilii muscle
Procerus muscle

Antagonists
Levator palpebrae superioris muscle
Tarsalis superior and inferior muscles
Epicranius muscle, frontal part

Innervation
Temporal and zygomatic branches of the facial nerve (cranial nerve VII)

5

5

Planning of treatment

The goal of the botulinum toxin treatment is to increase the vertical size of the palpebral aperture, creating the "open-eye look." The botulinum toxin injection widens the palpebral aperture and smoothes the skin of the lower eyelid.

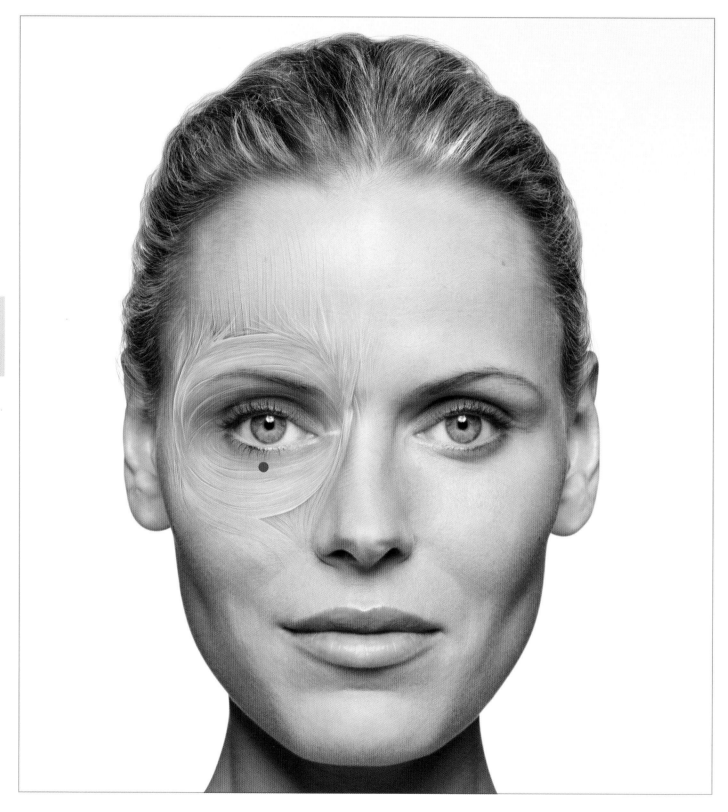

Treatment regimen

The injection of botulinum toxin type A should be given pretarsally, at a point along the midpupillar line, inserting the needle vertically and very superficially into the orbicularis oculi muscle.

⚠ Please observe the off-label therapy warnings relating to the licensed products (cf. section 1.12, p. 8) and the relevant product inserts.

Treatment

Injection

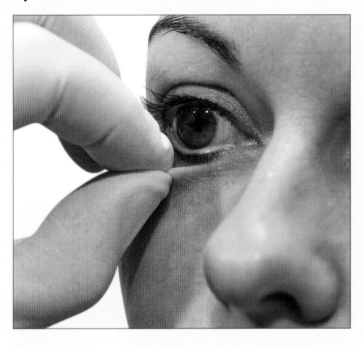

Snap-back test
The practitioner tests tissue elasticity and turgor with the snap-back test (cf. section 3.3, p. 24).

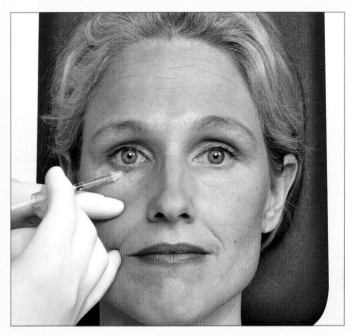

Injection technique
The injection is administered along the midpupillar line. The needle is inserted into the muscle vertically and very superficially.

Products and doses

Injection site	Product	Units/point	Ml solution/point
Pretarsal part of the orbicularis oculi muscle	Xeomin	1–2	0.025–0.05*
	Botox	1–2	0.025–0.05*
	Dysport	2.5–5	0.0125–0.025

Table 5.8 The authors' consensus dose recommendations for widening the palpebral aperture. The same data apply for products with identical substance preparations.
* Warning: If more than one unit is administered, it may be prudent to halve the dilution, i.e. administer a concentrated solution to reduce the risk of diffusion.

Correction factor
Man with active expressions: Factor 2
Age / inactive expressions: Factor 0.5.

Combined treatment options
Very suitable in combination with subsurfacing (fractional photothermolysis) or fractional laser resurfacing (e.g. Fraxel repair), provided that an experienced physician performs the procedure. The authors administer botulinum toxin prior to the other scheduled treatment measures.

Complications / Managing complications

A snap-back test (cf. Chapter 3.3, p. 24) is done before the injection. This allows the turgor and elasticity of the skin of the lower eyelids to be assessed. Slow or delayed skin retraction represents a contraindication to the injection. Undesirable enhancement of the fine lines may occur due to compensatory hyperactivation of the remaining orbicularis muscle fibers medially and laterally of the injection site.

Rarely, lymphedema may result due to the decreased pumping mechanism of the orbicularis oculi muscle. Excessive blockade of the palpebral region can lead to insufficient eye closure, impairment of the blinking reflex, reduced tear secretion and consequent drying of the cornea. Injections too far laterally may lead to ectropion of the lower eyelid and rounding of the lateral canthus.

Injections too far medially of the midpupillar line can cause reduced tear secretion and a dry eye. Weakening of the tone of the orbicularis oculi muscle can cause pseudohernias, i.e. the bags in the lower eyelids often associated with tear troughs. This situation can be aggravated by the administration of BTX-A, causing the face to look tired. Therefore, BTX-A should only be administered with caution to patients with pronounced tear troughs.

5

5.8 Bunny lines (nasal lines) | Nasalis muscle

Findings evaluation

Bunny lines are fine wrinkles of varying depth on the upper and lateral side of the wings of the nose. They may either be limited to the nose or radiate right up to the suborbital regions. These lines are produced by laughing and smiling, and are regarded as laughter lines. They do not occur with facial expressions that have a negative connotation, but are associated with positively motivated ones, giving the face a pleasant, even "cute" look.

Bunny lines may occur following treatment of the glabellar or orbital region, resulting from compensatory activation when blinking or squinting of the eyes. This situation is often an indication that the patient has been treated with botulinum toxin and should be avoided as much as possible.

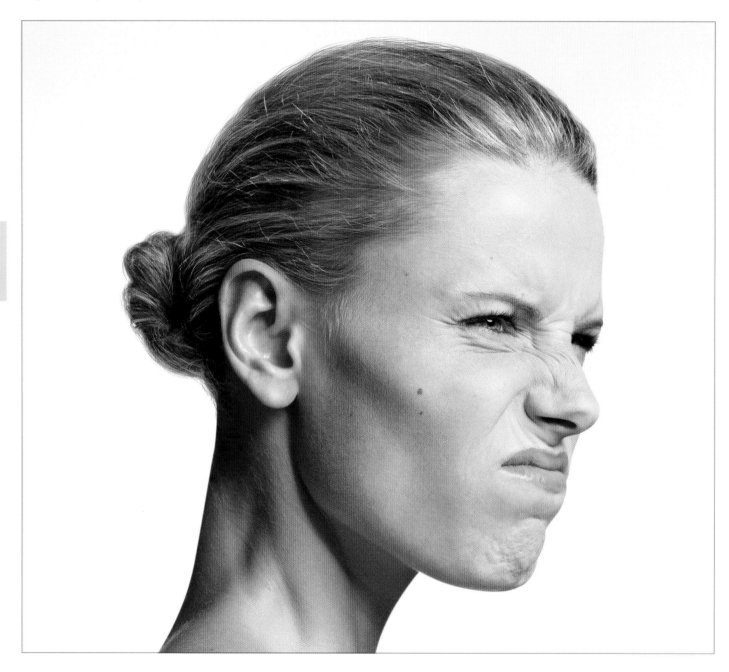

Patient selection

If the lines occur following treatment of the glabella and orbital region, they can be treated satisfactorily with very low doses of botulinum toxin in a follow-up treatment.
If nasal lines are already visible before the glabellar and/or orbital region is treated, they can also be treated directly during the same session.

If seen as cosmetically undesirable, nasal lines can also be treated in isolation.

Assessing the indication

With good patient selection, well suited for the smoothing of lines in the upper third of the nose.

⚠ Please observe the off-label therapy warnings relating to the licensed products (cf. section 1.12, p. 8) and the relevant product inserts.

Anatomy

The nasalis is the most important muscle involved in producing the bunny lines, and is also the target muscle when treating unwanted nasal lines. The following muscles act on the nose: nasalis, depressor septi nasi, levator labii superioris alaeque nasi and procerus muscles (cf. section 5.2, p. 46 ff.).

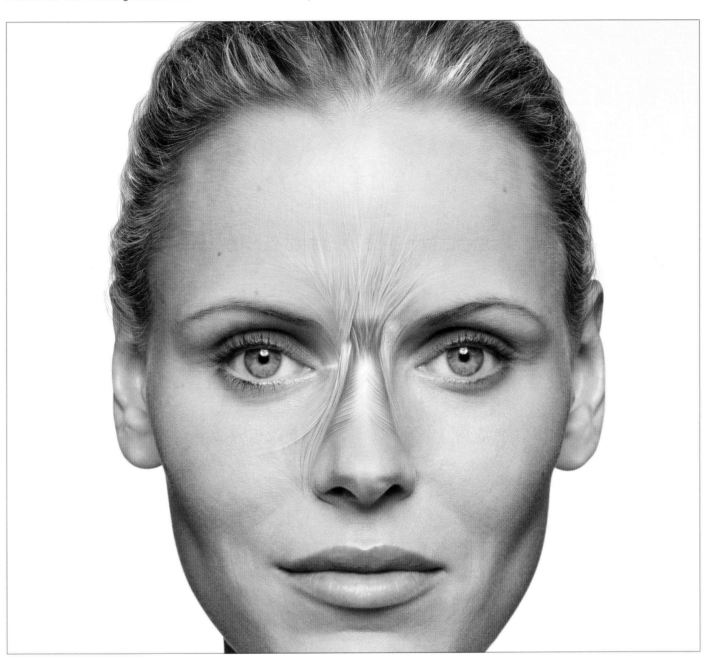

Origin
Alveolar jugum of the lateral incisor and the canine

Insertion
Wing of the nose at the margin of the nostril
Lateral nasal cartilage
Aponeurosis of the dorsum of the nose

Function
Upper (alar) part: dilates the nostrils
Lower, transverse parts of the muscle: compresses the nostrils and pulls the tip of the nose slightly downwards

Synergists
Levator labii superioris alaeque nasi muscle
Depressor septi nasi muscle

Antagonists
None

Innervation
Buccal branches of the facial nerve (cranial nerve VII)

Planning of treatment

The treatment goal is to reduce the nasal lines referred to as bunny lines. These fine lines occuring lateral of the nose bridge can develop either naturally or following treatment with botulinum toxin of the glabella or lateral canthal region.

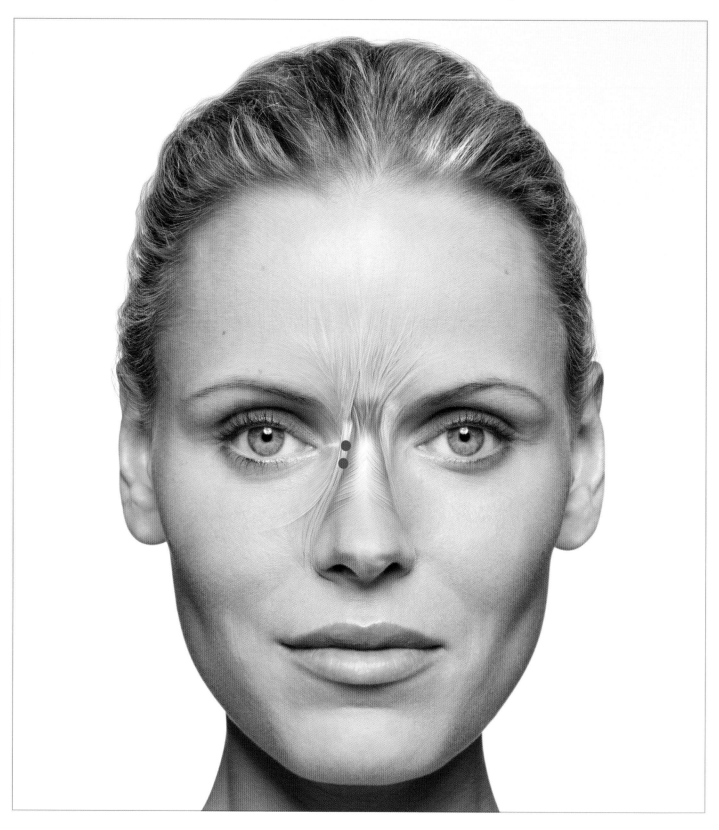

Treatment regimen

Nasal lines are treated with an injection of botulinum toxin A, administered into one to two points (depending on line breadth) per side in the middle, upper part of the wing of the nose. The needle should be inserted superficially.

⚠ Please observe the off-label therapy warnings relating to the licensed products (cf. section 1.12, p. 8) and the relevant product inserts.

Treatment

Injection

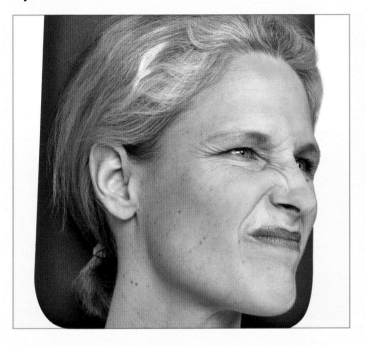

Activation
The practitioner instructs the patient to contract the muscle actively: "Squint your eyes as if you were looking into the sun without your sunglasses."

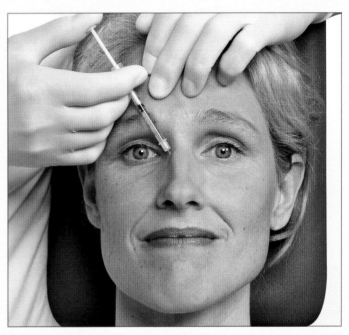

Injection technique.
The needle is inserted flat or at an angle of no greater than 45 degrees to the skin, to avoid contact with the periosteum, which is highly sensitive to pain. The injection is given using the intradermal wheal technique.

5

Products and doses

Injection site	Product	Units/point	Ml solution/point
Nasalis muscle	**Xeomin**	1	0.025
	Botox	1	0.025
	Dysport	2.5	0.0125

Table 5.9 The authors' consensus dose recommendations for the treatment of bunny lines. The same data apply for products with identical substance preparations.

Correction factor

Man with active expressions: Factor 2
Age / inactive expressions: Factor 0.5.

Combined treatment options

Very suitable in combination with percutaneous collagen induction, subsurfacing (fractional photothermolysis) or fractional laser resurfacing (e.g. Fraxel repair), provided that the procedure is performed by an experienced physician. The authors administer botulinum toxin prior to the other scheduled treatment measures.

 Complications / Managing complications

Small hematomas may develop at the puncture site. Slight bleeding can be controlled by compression with a Q-tip (cotton bud). The injection should not be given too far laterally of the wings of the nose. This carries the risk of blockade of the levator labii superioris alaeque nasi muscle, which may lead to ptosis of the upper lip, impairing speech and closure of the mouth.
In theory, double vision may occur due to unintended, diffusion-related blockade of the rectus inferioris or medialis muscle.

5.9 Gummy smile | Levator labii superioris muscle

Findings evaluation

The upper lip is pulled too far upwards when a person laughs or smiles, with disproportionate exposure of the teeth and gums. Those affected often find this "gummy smile" cosmetically undesirable. This smile pattern is also frequently associated with deep nasolabial lines.

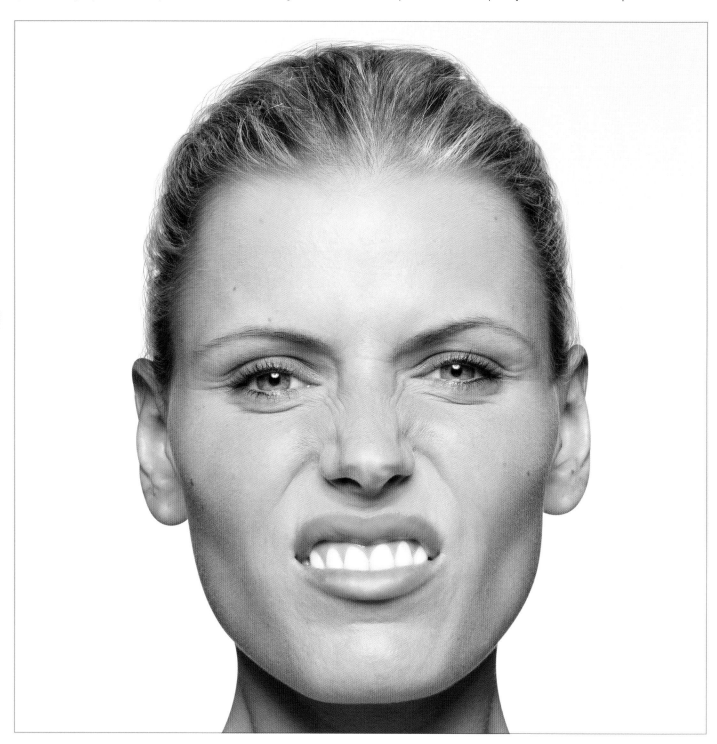

Patient selection

The evaluation is carried out at rest and under dynamic conditions. At rest, people with a gummy smile tend to have a narrow upper lip and their upper incisors are visible. When they smile, the gums are clearly visible while the upper lip becomes thinner and may even be slightly inverted.

Assessing the indication

The potential interactions of the muscles in the perioral region are highly complex, so that a good treatment result depends on three key factors, namely the therapist's experience, optimum patient selection and the correct dose and placement. In general, this indication is the preserve of therapists with experience in this specialist area.

⚠ Please observe the off-label therapy warnings relating to the licensed products (cf. section 1.12, p. 8) and the relevant product inserts.

Anatomy

Hyperactivity of the levator labii superioris muscle is one factor that produces the gummy smile. Another is the involvement of the levator labii superioris alaeque nasi muscle, since it lifts the medial part of the upper lip when it contracts.

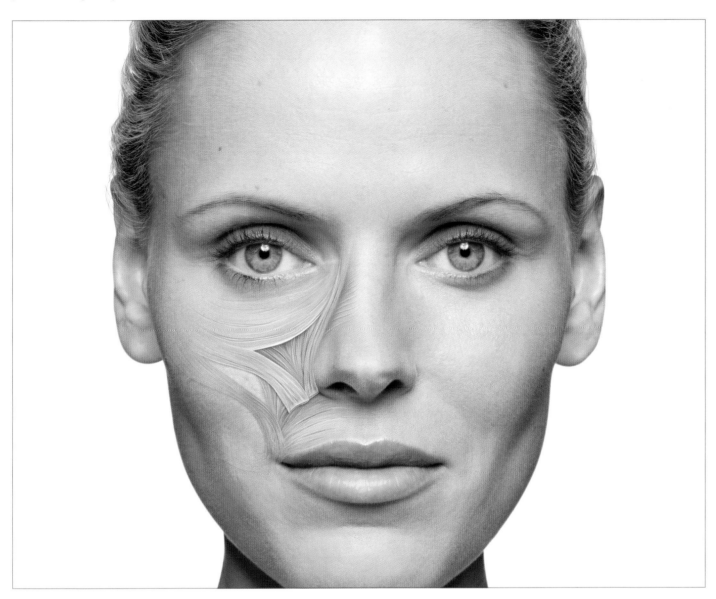

Levator labii superioris muscle					
Origin	**Insertion**	**Function**	**Synergists**	**Antagonists**	**Innervation**
Infraorbital margin of the maxilla Zygomatic bone	Radiates into the fibers of the orbicularis oris muscle Skin of the upper lip	Lifts the upper lip and deepens the nasolabial lines	Levator labii superioris alaeque nasi muscle (lateral parts)	Depressor anguli oris muscle Orbicularis oris muscle	Temporal branches of the facial nerve (cranial nerve VII)

Levator labii superioris alaeque nasi muscle					
Frontal process of the maxilla Muscle mass of the orbicularis oculi muscle	Wings of the nose Upper lip Lateral and dorsal circumference of the nostril	Lifts the upper lip (together with the other levators) Lifts the free edge of the nostrils and stops the wings of the nose from collapsing	Levator labii superioris nasalis muscle Zygomaticus major and minor muscles Levator anguli oris muscle	Depressor anguli oris muscle Orbicularis oris muscle	Zygomatic branches of the facial nerve (cranial nerve VII)

Table 5.10 Both muscles are involved in producing the gummy smile.

Planning of treatment

The treatment goal consists of reducing the hyperactivity of the muscles responsible for the gummy smile and to reduce the amount of gum exposure. Weakening these muscles makes the smile more harmonious and pleasing to the eye.

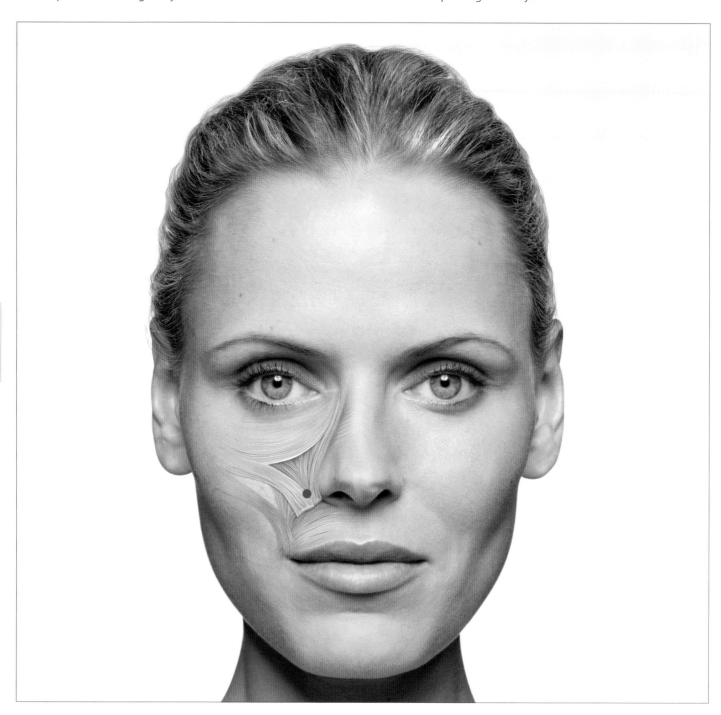

Practical tip

The injection regimen is dependent on whether or not the gummy smile is associated with deepening of the nasolabial lines. This is assessed by asking the patient to smile as widely as possible.

Treatment regimen

If the gummy smile occurs without the formation of nasolabial lines, the injection is sited slightly further down in the region of the levator labii superioris muscle. This injection is deeper: the needle should penetrate the more superficial orbicularis oris muscle to reach the underlying fibers of the levator labii superioris alaeque nasi and levator labii superioris muscles.

If the exposure of the maxillary incisors is associated with deepening of the nasolabial lines, the injection is given into the labial part of the levator labii superioris alaeque nasi muscle, inserting the needle into the bulge at the uppermost segment of the nasolabial line. At this level, the muscle is very superficially located, and the maximum injection depth should therefore be 3 mm.

⚠ Please observe the off-label therapy warnings relating to the licensed products (cf. section 1.12, p. 8) and the relevant product inserts.

Treatment

Injection

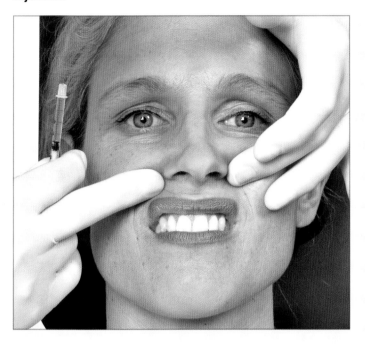

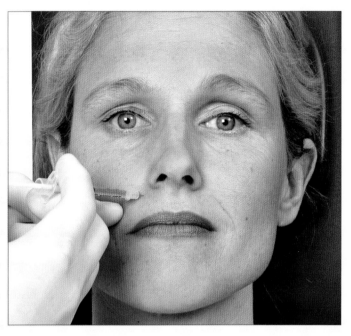

Activation
The practitioner instructs the patient to contract the muscle actively: "Smile as widely as possible."

Injection technique
Injected directed into the center of maximum contraction in the caudal part of the levator labii superioris muscle: the needle penetrates through the more superficial orbicularis oris muscle to reach the underlying fibers of the levator labii superioris alaeque nasi and levator labii superioris muscles.

5

Products and doses

Injection site	Product	Units/point	Ml solution/point
Levator labii superioris (alaeque nasi) muscles	Xeomin	1	0.025
	Botox	1	0.025
	Dysport	2.5	0.0125

Table 5.11 The authors' consensus dose recommendations for the treatment of a gummy smile. The same data apply for products with identical substance preparations.

Correction factor

Man with active expressions: Factor 2
Age / inactive expressions: Factor 0.5.

 Complications / Managing complications

Asymmetry is one of the most common complications. This generally does not manifest at rest, but only during active function, i.e. when smiling or laughing. Milder asymmetry is tolerable or can be corrected at the patient's request, but any major asymmetry should be remedied immediately. Dose titration is advisable: first give about half the planned dose, assess the effect after 2 weeks, then administer the rest. Documentation of the baseline findings and the treatment result provides an objective measure of the extent of any asymmetry.
More potent weakening of the muscle causes the medial part of the upper lip to droop. This can lead to a compensatory intensification of the activity of the zygomaticus major muscle. The more lateral pull causes widening of the oral aperture, known as the "Joker" smile. This can be balanced out with mild blockade of the zygomaticus major muscle.

5.10 Lines around the upper and lower lip | Orbicularis oris muscle

Findings evaluation

Radial, i.e. ray-like lines around the upper and lower lip are a visible sign of aging. The subcutis of the upper lip is very thin. This, together with the pronounced activity of the orbicularis oris muscle, results in a particular predisposition to lines in this region.

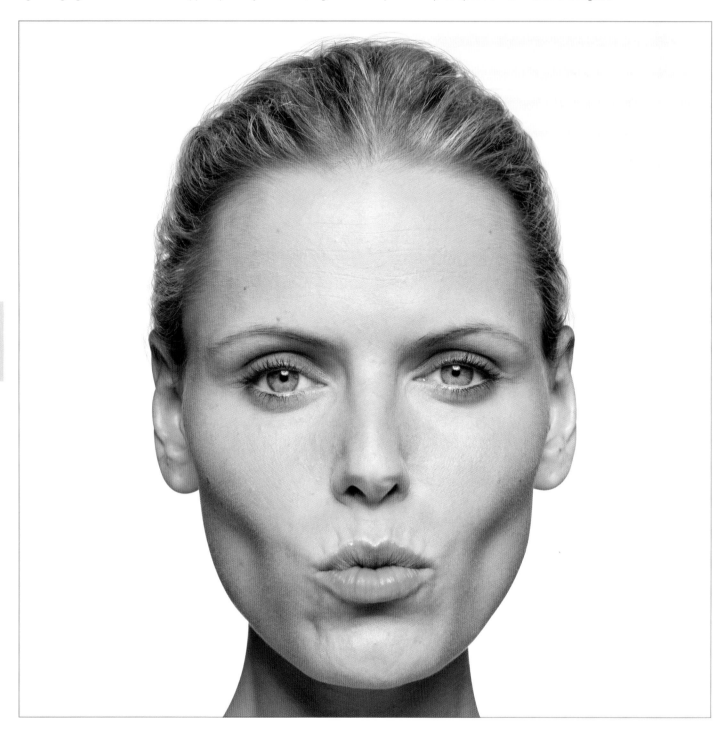

Patient selection

Since the mouth region is typically treated only with very low doses, there are limits to the effects that can be expected. Patients should be warned about this. The consequences of temporary partial insufficiency of the orbicularis oris muscle should also be mentioned during the pre-treatment information session. Professional musicians who play wind instruments should only be treated with botulinum toxin with extreme caution in the region around the mouth.

Early treatment of the upper lip may be considered as a way of preventing lines in younger women.

Assessing the indication

Treatment of the lips tends to be a second-line indication for botulinum toxin, used to optimize augmentation with hyaluronic acid.

⚠ Please observe the off-label therapy warnings relating to the licensed products (cf. section 1.12, p. 8) and the relevant product inserts.

Anatomy

The orbicularis oris muscle provides the basis of the motor apparatus of the lips. The section of the muscular ring that lies furthest from the oral aperture can reduce its size while protruding the red margin of the lips, as when whistling. If the part that lies at the edge of the lips (within the red margin) contracts in isolation, the red margin inclines towards the front teeth, so that less of it is visible. The tone of this muscle is important in retaining saliva, which is discharged from the angle of the mouth if the muscle is paralyzed.

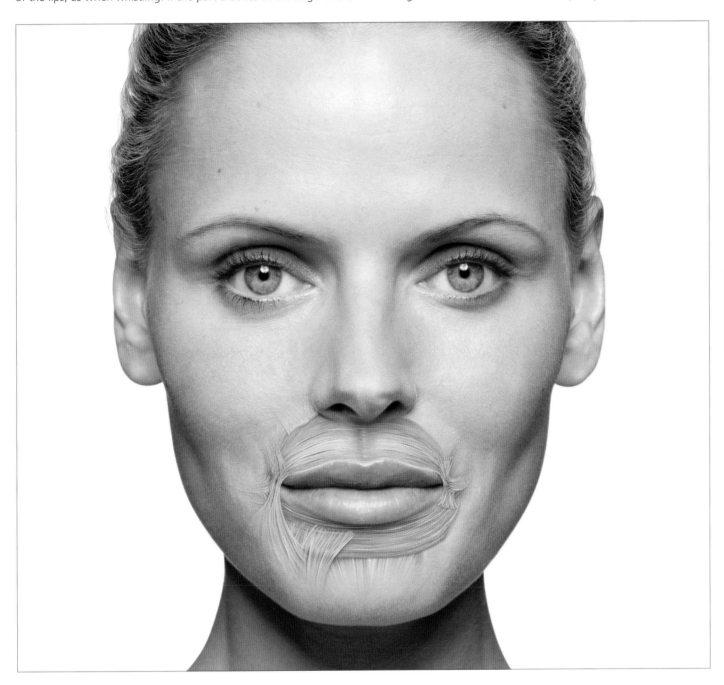

5

Origin
Mandible
Maxilla

Insertion
Upper and lower lip

Function
Closes the lips
Purses the lips as when kissing or whistling

Antagonists
All the facial expression muscles which pull the lips or the angle of the mouth in the lateral direction, upwards or downwards, thus widening the oral aperture, act as antagonists

Innervation
Buccal branches and marginal mandibular branch of the facial nerve (cranial nerve VII)

Planning of treatment

The goal of the botulinum toxin injection treatment is to reduce or remove the radial lines around the upper and lower lip. Very small doses are indicated in order to avoid possible problems in mouth closing. Moreover, low-level botulinum toxin treatment of the upper and lower lip can also be proper for wrinkle prevention.

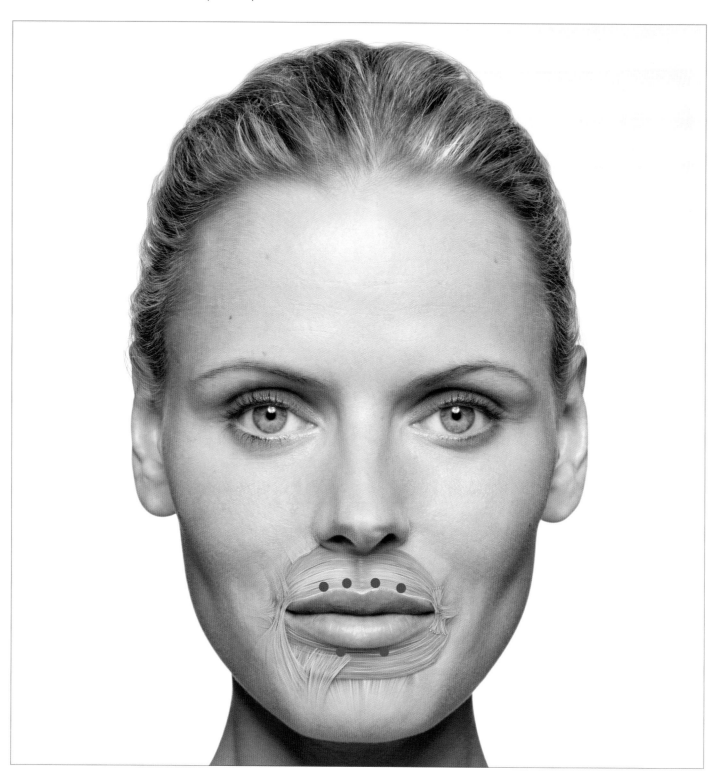

Practical tip

The focus is on the treatment of the central lines close to philtrum. The lateral lines are better treated with augmentation procedures due to the risk of insufficient mouth closure if botulinum toxin is used.

Treatment regimen

The injection points are located at the bases of the lines, where the red margin of the lips meets the normal skin, and are dependent on the relief of the lines.

⚠ Please observe the off-label therapy warnings relating to the licensed products (cf. section 1.12, p. 8) and the relevant product inserts.

Treatment

Injection

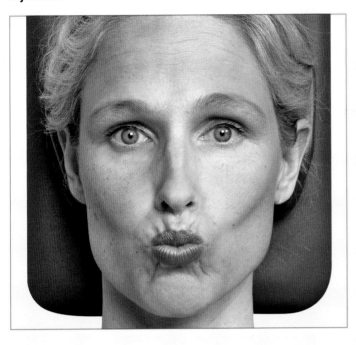

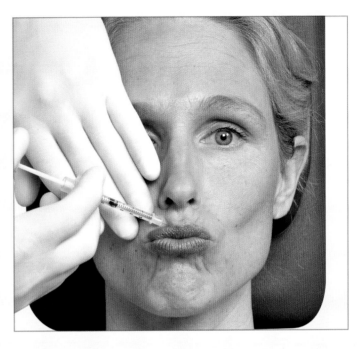

5

Activation
The practitioner instructs the patient to contract the muscle actively: "Purse your lips as if you are going to whistle."

Injection technique
Cooling of the upper lip before the treatment is advisable, as the injections can be painful. The injection is given subcutaneously, directly at the base of each line where the red margin of the lips meets the normal skin.

Products and doses

Injection site	Product	Units/point	Ml solution/point
Orbicularis oris muscle	Xeomin	0.5	0.0125
	Botox	0.5	0.0125
	Dysport	1.25	0.00625

Table 5.12 The authors' consensus dose recommendations for the treatment of lines around the upper lip. The same data apply for products with identical substance preparations.

Correction factor
Man with active expressions: Factor 1.5
Age / inactive expressions: Factor 0.5.

Combined treatment options
The upper and lower lip regions are typical indications for augmentation therapy and ideal candidates for a combined treatment of filler injections restoring volume and shape, with botulinum toxin therapy damping active wrinkle formation. Optimally suitable is also the combination with percutaneous collagen induction therapy achieving natural improvement of the very fine wrinkles without giving risk of complications or side-effects in this vulnerable region.

Complications / Managing complications

Overtreatment leads to functional impairment with insufficient mouth closure, articulation problems and difficulties with eating and drinking. Therefore, this area is typically treated with very low doses.

5.11 Marionette lines | Depressor anguli oris muscle

Findings evaluation

The marionette lines start from the corners of the mouth and continue down to the chin. Pronounced lines of this type give the face a frustrated, disappointed or dissatisfied expression. Drooping at the corners of the mouth is one of the most powerful negative messages communicated by the face, second only to the frown line. The depressor anguli oris (also called the triangularis) is the key muscle involved in the intensity of these lines.

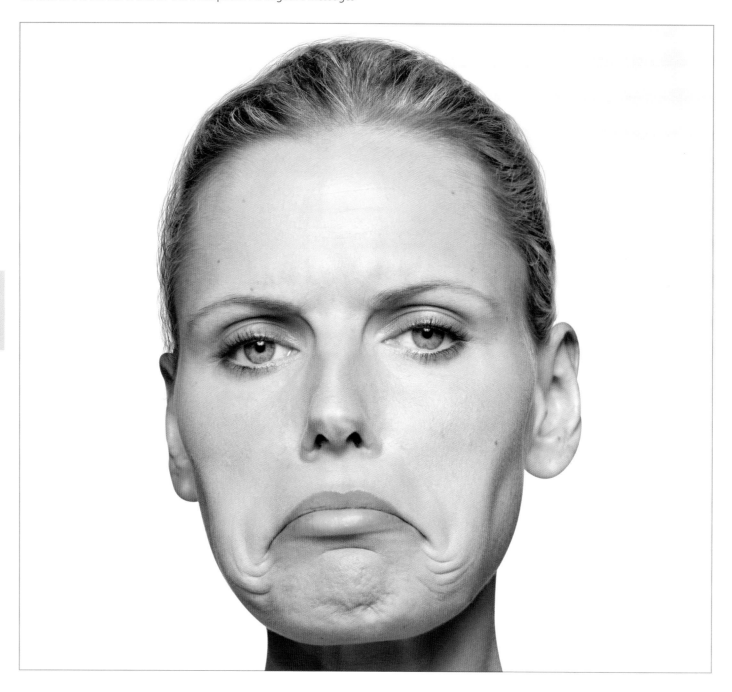

Patient selection

Patients who can produce or intensify these lines dynamically and voluntarily benefit from the treatment. That means kinetic and hyperkinetic patients (cf. section 3.4, p. 25 f.) are the most suitable. Patients whose marionette lines are caused by aged-related subcutaneous tissue atrophy, i.e. ptosis of the SMAS (superficial musculo-aponeurotic system)or skin excess are less suited for treatment with botulinum toxin. These patients are usually better treated with augmentation procedures and if necessary surgery.

Assessing the indication

Marionette lines are regarded as a strong indication for treatment with botulinum toxin A. However, this procedure should always be combined with augmentation methods acting against the age-related changes in facial soft-tissues primarily involved in the formation of marionette lines.

⚠ Please observe the off-label therapy warnings relating to the licensed products (cf. section 1.12, p. 8) and the relevant product inserts.

Anatomy

The perioral muscles are in several layers. The depressor anguli oris muscle is the most superficial muscle in the chin region. When it contracts, this muscle pulls down the angle of the mouth together with offshoots of the platysma, giving the face the frustrated, disappointed or dissatisfied expression mentioned at the beginning of this section.

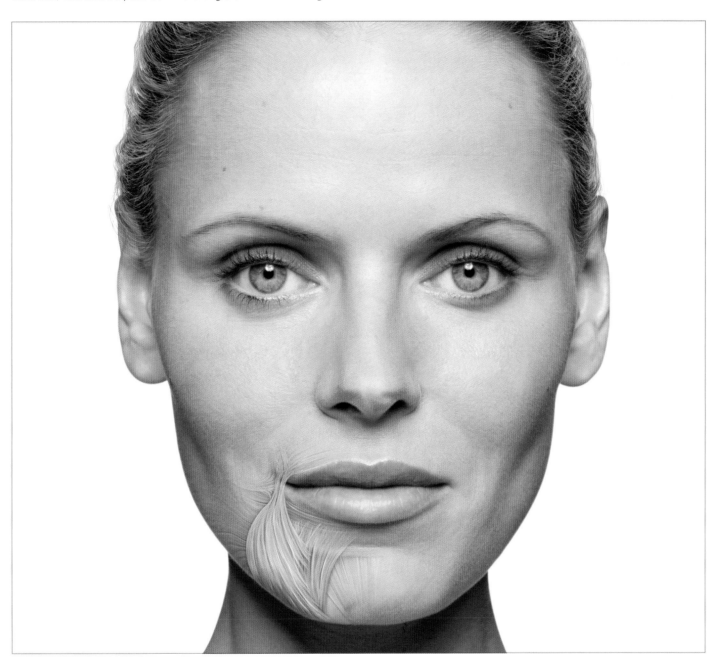

5

Origin
Lower edge of the mandible, caudal of the mental foramen

Insertion
Angle of the mouth, cheek

Function
Pulls the angle of the mouth and the platysma downwards

Synergists
Platysma
Depressor labii inferioris muscle

Antagonists
Zygomaticus major muscle
Levator anguli oris muscle

Innervation
Marginal mandibular branch of the facial nerve (cranial nerve VII)

5

Planning of treatment

The goal of the treatment with botulinum toxin A is to raise the lowered angle of the mouth at rest. This is achieved by a dose-dependent reduction in tone of the depressor anguli oris muscle and the corresponding overlying segments of the platysma.

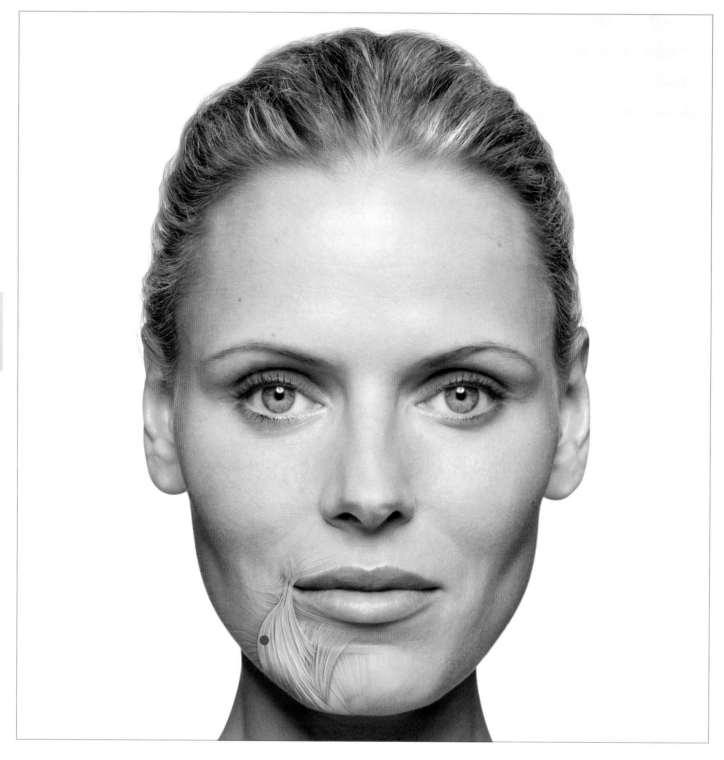

Practical tip

Both the depressor anguli oris muscle and the fibers of the platysma can be rendered visible and palpable if contracted.

The closer to the labial angle the injection, the more effective it is, though with a concomitant increase in the risk of undesirable diffusion into the muscles of the mouth region.

Treatment regimen

A deep injection is used, given well laterally of the marionette lines, so as to include the cranial parts of the platysma. The injection site should be at least 1 cm lower than the angle of the mouth, to avoid diffusion into the orbicularis oris muscle.

⚠ Please observe the off-label therapy warnings relating to the licensed products (cf. section 1.12, p. 8) and the relevant product inserts.

Treatment

Injection

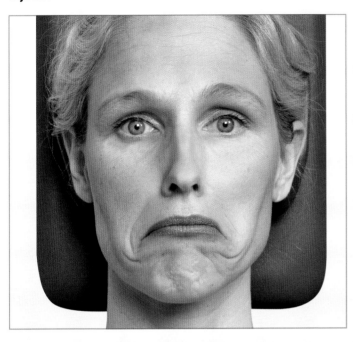

Activation
The practitioner instructs the patient to contract the muscle actively: "Pull the corners of your mouth downwards."

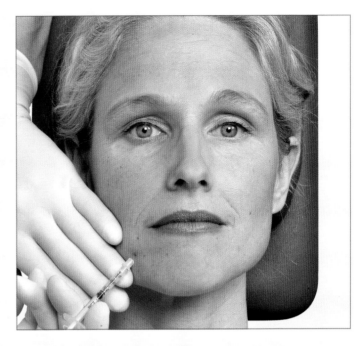

Injection technique
The injection point is located lateral of the marionette line. The needle is inserted almost vertically, directly into the middle to caudal part of the muscle, also infiltrating the cranial segments of the platysma.

5

Products and doses

Injection site	Product	Units/point	Ml solution/point
Depressor anguli oris muscle	**Xeomin**	2–3	0.05–0.075
	Botox	2–3	0.05–0.075
	Dysport	5–7.5	0.025–0.0375

Table 5.13 The authors' consensus dose recommendations for the treatment of marionette lines. The same data apply for products with identical substance preparations.

Correction factor
Man with active expressions: Factor 1.5
Age / inactive expressions: Factor 0.5.

Combined treatment options
This treatment of marionette lines makes for an excellent combination with various augmentation methods increasing tissue density, stabilization and filling of volume. Rather than as an option to supplement, augmentation therapy should be regarded as the first way to go for this indication, suitable in combination with botulinum toxin A if muscular activity is involved in the formation of the marionette lines.

Complications / Managing complications

Diffusion into the depressor labii inferioris muscle leads to asymmetric lower lip configuration.
Over-treatment and/or an injection given too close to the angle of the mouth can lead to functional impairment in the form of insufficient mouth closure, with results that may include problems or asymmetries of eating, drinking and speech.

5.12 Cobblestone chin | Mentalis muscle

Findings evaluation

Intense contraction of the mentalis muscle leads to uneven, irregular wrinkling of the skin surface of the chin reminding of a cobblestone-like pattern. In some cases, this can also occur when the person speaks, appearing in sudden, brief flashes.

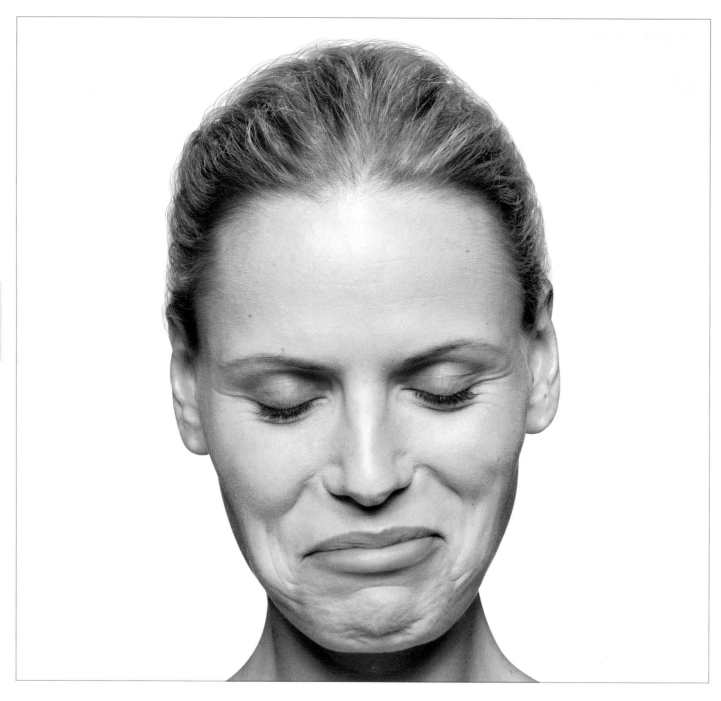

Patient selection / Assessing the indication

Treatment of a cobblestone chin is usually done in combination with other facial rejuvenation procedures. The irregularities in the relief of the chin, produced by muscle activity, can generally be treated with good results. A cobblestone chin becomes particularly noticeable following treatment of the forehead or the glabella, as the chin would not previously have been a conspicuous feature in a hyperkinetically active face.

⚠ Please observe the off-label therapy warnings relating to the licensed products (cf. section 1.12, p. 8) and the relevant product inserts.

Anatomy

Intermittent, cobblestone-like contours on the chin develop due to increased activitiy of the mentalis muscle combined with age-related subcutaneous fat atrophy. This is further related to advancing sla-cking of the mandibular and submental retaining ligaments seen with age.

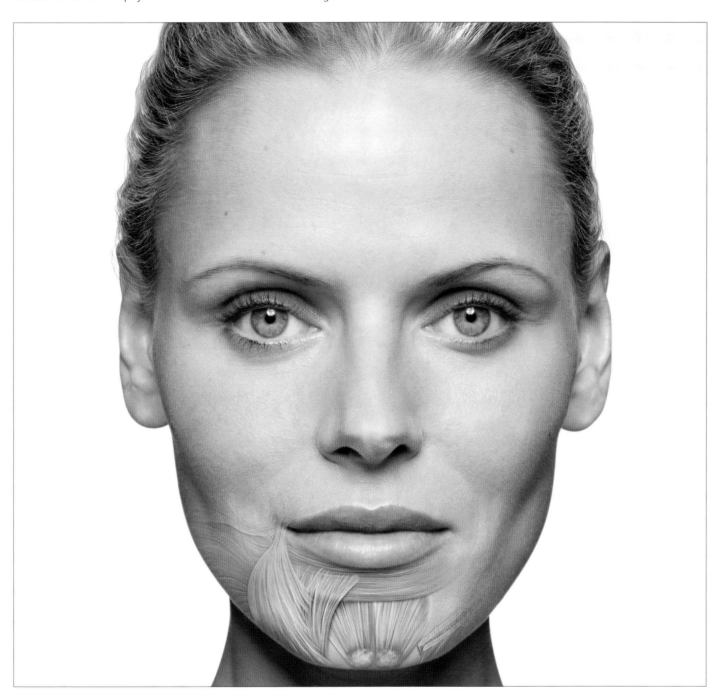

5

Origin
Mandible, alveolar jugum of the lateral incisor

Insertion
Radiates into the skin of the chin

Function
Involved in pushing up the central lower lip, often leading to a de-pression of the lateral lower lip

Synergists
Depressor labii inferioris muscle
Depressor anguli oris muscle

Antagonists
Zygomaticus major muscle
Levator anguli oris muscle

Innervation
Facial nerve (cranial nerve VII)

Planning of treatment

The goal of the botulinum toxin type A treatment is a dose-dependent relaxation of the mentalis muscle. The damped muscular activity will lead to smoothing of the skin at the tip of the chin during natural facial expressions. The appearance of a cobblestone chin thus can be reduced or prevented.

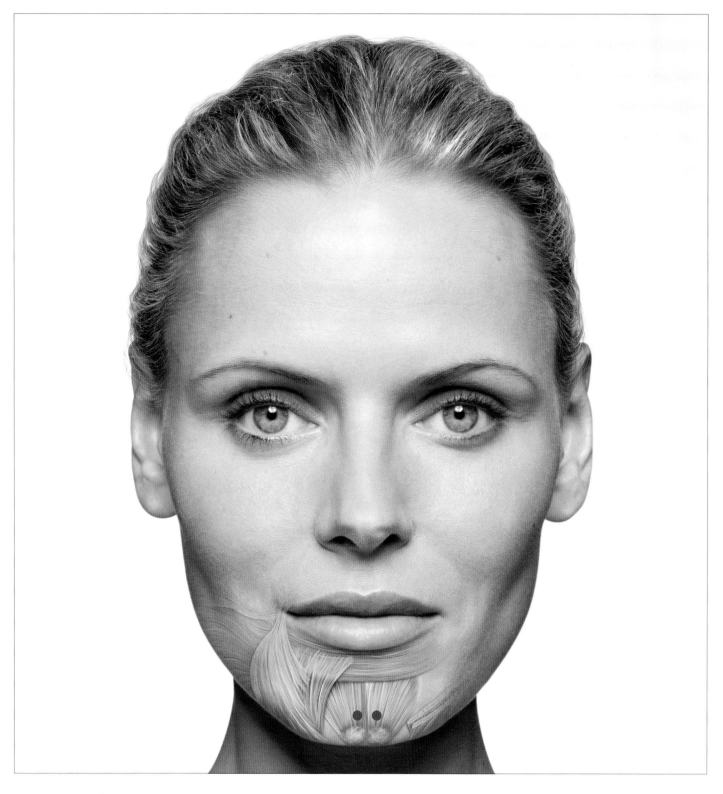

Treatment regimen

One injection each is given on the right and left side, directly into the relevant muscle segments. A minimum distance of 3 cm from the lower lip is maintained, to avoid unwanted co-treatment of the orbicularis oris muscle. The injection points should also be placed as close as possible to the median line to avoid diffusion into the depressor labii inferioris muscle.

⚠ Please observe the off-label therapy warnings relating to the licensed products (cf. section 1.12, p. 8) and the relevant product inserts.

Treatment

Injection

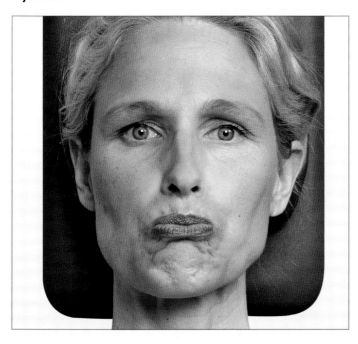

Activation
The practitioner instructs the patient to contract the muscle actively: "Push up your lower lip."

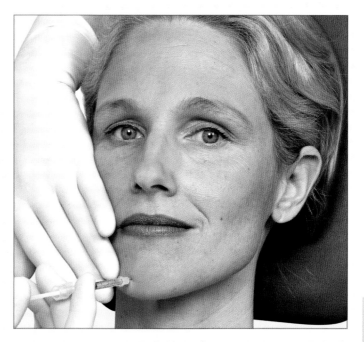

Injection technique
The needle is inserted perpendicularly to the skin, directly into each muscle belly, administering one injection per belly.

Products and doses

Injection site	Product	Units/point	Ml solution/point
Mentalis muscle	**Xeomin**	2–3	0.05–0.075
	Botox	2–3	0.05–0.075
	Dysport	5–7.5	0.025–0.0375

Table 5.14 The authors' consensus dose recommendations for the treatment of cobblestone chin. The same data apply for products with identical substance preparations.

Correction factor
Man with active expressions: Factor 1.5
Age / inactive expressions: Factor 0.5.

Combined treatment options
The treatment of cobblestone chin can be combined with various augmentation procedures.

 Complications / Managing complications

The risk of complications with this injection technique is low but potentially a serious one. Functional impairment in the form of insufficient mouth closure may result from the loss of support to the soft tissues of the lower face. These untoward results stem from a loss of oral competence and may include problems or asymmetries of eating, drinking and speech. For these reasons an initial lower dose, avoiding the surrounding muscles (unless they are intended targets), and leaving enough mentalis strength to support the lower face are key.

5

5.13 Bruxism | Masseter muscle

Findings evaluation

Bruxism or teeth grinding is physically caused by repetitive, unconscious contraction of the masseter muscle. Most people occasionally grind or clench their teeth, generally not causing harm. However, when bruxism occurs on a regular basis, typically during sleep, it can lead to damage and oral health complications and therefore becomes a medical as well as an aesthetic problem. Hypertrophy of the masseter muscle further occurs frequently in men leading to the characteristic appearance of a massive, edged mandible. Those affected are often bothered about the severity and unintended aggressive expression that emanates from their facial features. For that reason, hypertrophy of the masseter muscle even regardless of occurring bruxism is a common aesthetic indication nowadays , especially in Asia.

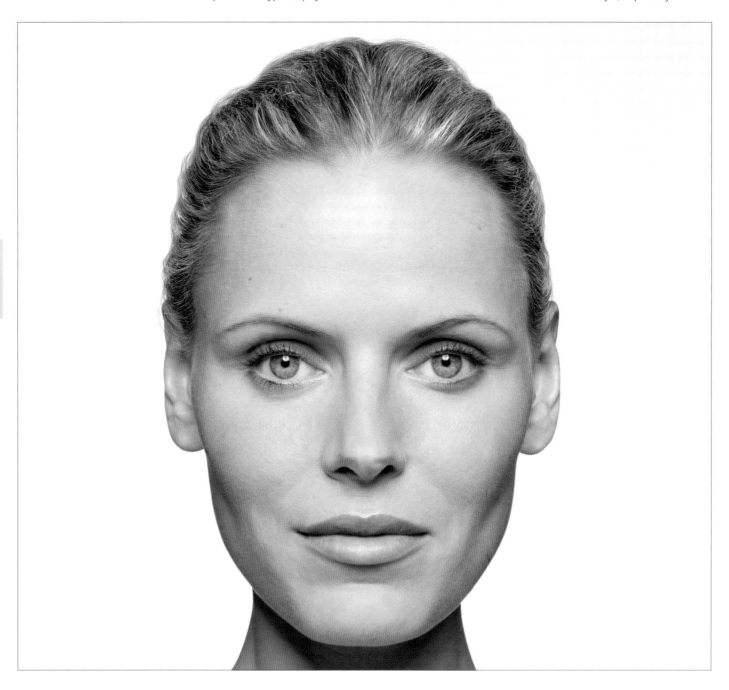

Patient selection/ Assessing the indication

The etiology of bruxism can be varied and so there are various therapeutic strategies. A dose-dependent relaxation of the masseter muscle with botulinum toxin A can be considered as a suitable treatment option for mild to more severe cases of bruxism. However, if bruxism is associated with mental stress, further psychological approaches are to be recommended in any case.

Given a mere aesthetic need, treatment with botulinum toxin A is a promising method to soften the appearance of a pronounced jaw–chin area, especially frequently needed in men, and a gentle alternative to surgery.

⚠ Please observe the off-label therapy warnings relating to the licensed products (cf. section 1.12, p. 8) and the relevant product inserts.

Anatomy

The Masseter belongs to the masticatory muscles and has its function in closing the mandibular jaw onto the maxillary jaw. Synergistically working with the temporal muscle and taking turns in contracting with the lateral pterygoid muscle, the superficial and deep portion of the Masseter facilitate the grinding movement of the mandibular jaw.

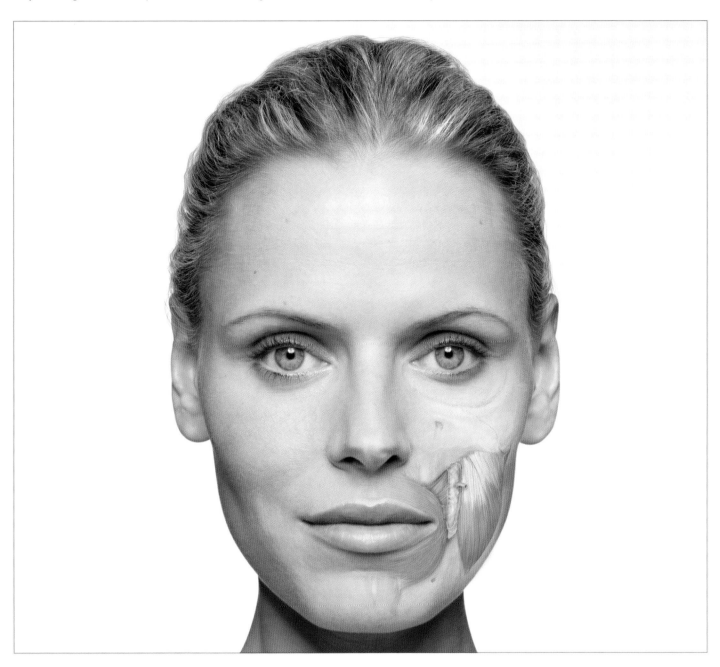

Origin
Superficial portion: Zygomatic process of the maxilla and lower border of the zygomatic arch
Deep portion: Posterior 3rd of the lower border and whole of the medial surface of the zygomatic arch

Insertion
Superficial portion: Angle and lower half of the lateral surface of the ramus of the mandible
Deep portion: Upper half of the ramus and lateral surface of the coronoid process of the mandible

Function
Lifting the mandibular jaw, jaw occlusion

Synergists
Temporal muscle, medial pterygoid muscle

Antagonists
Gravity, lateral pterygoid muscle (when contracted simultaneously on both sides)

Innervation
Mandibular division (V3) of the trigeminal nerve

93

Planning of treatment

The goal of the botulinum toxin A treatment is a dose-dependent relaxation of the masseter muscle. This can be either indicated to improve bruxism or to mellow the appearance of a prominent male jaw. The smoothed mandibular contours will provide the patient a more gentle, appealing look.

5

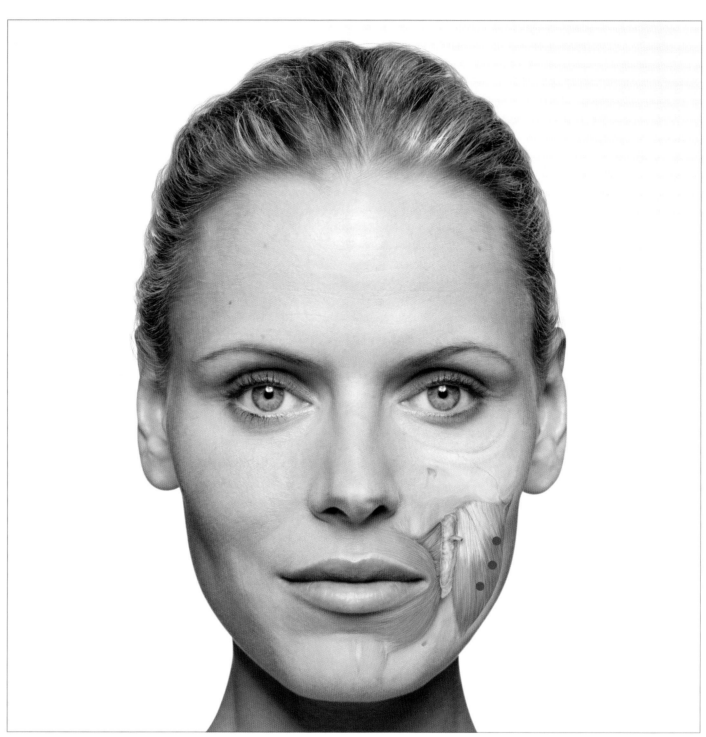

Practical tip

Dosing is dependent on whether the treatment has medical or aesthetic reasons, as well as on individual findings. Treatment of bruxism generally indicates higher substance doses than therapy in a mere aesthetic respect. Since visible hypertrophy of the masseter muscle primarily occurs in men, the consensus dose recommendations given below refer to men and should be reduced if adapted to women.

Treatment regimen

To treat bruxism, 5–6 injections can be given on the right and left into the deeper parts of the muscle using the direct technique. For aesthetic therapy, 3–4 injections per side are given in a triangular shape into the more superficial layers of the muscle's Punctum mobile.

⚠ Please observe the off-label therapy warnings relating to the licensed products (cf. section 1.12, p. 8) and the relevant product inserts.

Treatment

Injection

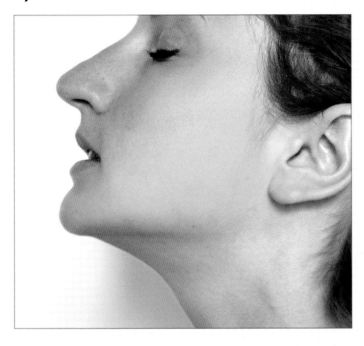

Activation
The practitioner instructs the patient to active contraction of the muscle: "Strongly clench your teeth."

Injection technique
The needle is inserted perpendicularly to the skin, directly injecting into the muscle belly at 3–4 sites in a triangular shape.

5

Products and doses

Injection site	Product	Units/point	Ml solution/point
Masseter muscle	**Xeomin**	2–4	0.05–0.1
	Botox	2–4	0.05-0.1
	Dysport	5–10	0.025–0.05

Table 5.15 The authors' consensus dose recommendations for the treatment of the masseter muscle. The same data apply for products with identical substance preparations.

Correction factor
Man with very pronounced masseter activity: Factor 1.5
Female / age :   Factor 0.5.

Combined treatment options
Aesthetic correction of the jaw can be combined with augmentation procedures and if requested surgery.

Complications / Managing complications

Over-treatment can lead to restricted masticatory function causing problems in chewing and eating. Further unwanted side effects due to unpredicted diffusion behavior is weakening the oral muscles of mastication or speaking as well as possible complications of the auditory system caused by diffusion into the ear region.

5.14 Platysmal bands | Platysma

Findings evaluation

Platysmal bands or cords become more pronounced with age. They stand out prominently when the facial expression muscles are used or when speaking. In some patients, and in particular in advanced years, the platysmal bands can be steadily apparent, impairing the person's overall appearance.

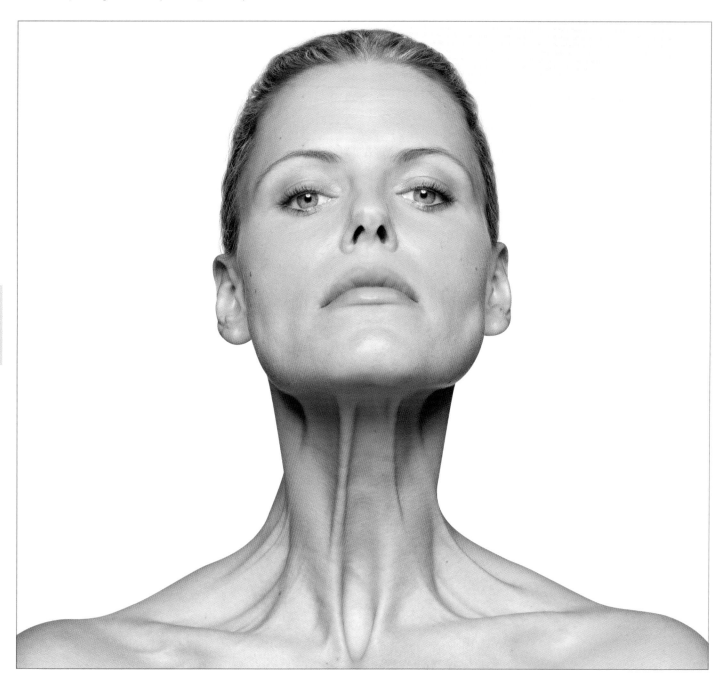

Patient selection

Individuals who contract the platysma voluntarily and can make the longitudinal bands or cords stand out will benefit most. In the preliminary consultation, it will be necessary to evaluate whether the patient has a history of cosmetic surgery, such as facelifts. During this discussion, the patient will need to be warned about the limitations of firming the neck with botulinum toxin, particularly the fact that the horizontal lines on the neck will not be influenced significantly with the procedure. One option that could be considered for these lines consists of augmentation methods using fillers.

A complete platysma treatment may involve a relatively high dose, as several cords typically occur and will need to be treated with the corresponding number of units of botulinum toxin.

Assessing the indication

A good and readily treatable indication if patient selection is good. Patients with a great deal of excess, lax skin in the neck are poor candidates.

⚠ Please observe the off-label therapy warnings relating to the licensed products (cf. section 1.12, p. 8) and the relevant product inserts.

Anatomy

As the cutaneous muscle of the neck, the platysma can tighten the skin of the anterior part of the neck from the lower jaw to the clavicles when contracted voluntarily – e.g. by pulling down both corners of the mouth. When this happens, its individual muscle cords often become visible through the skin.

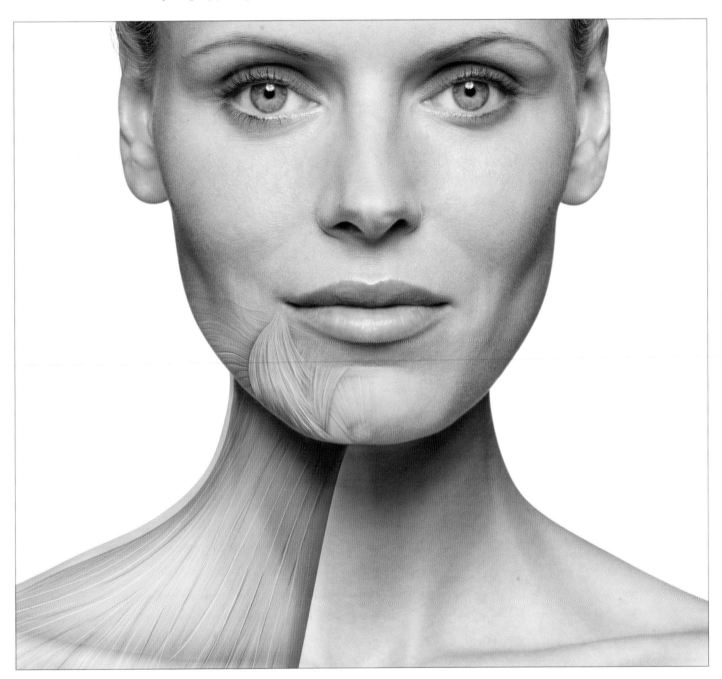

Origin
Base of the mandible
Parotid fascia

Insertion
Skin caudally of the clavicle
Pectoral fascia

Function
Helps pull down the corners of the mouth
Helps open the mouth

Synergists
Depressor anguli oris muscle

Antagonists
Levator anguli oris muscle

Innervation
Cervical branch of the facial nerve (cranial nerve VII)

Planning of treatment

The treatment goal of the therapy with botulinum toxin type A is a dose-dependent reduction of tone of the individual platysmal muscle cords. Treatment of the platysmal cords should also be considered in therapy of marionette lines with botulinum toxin.

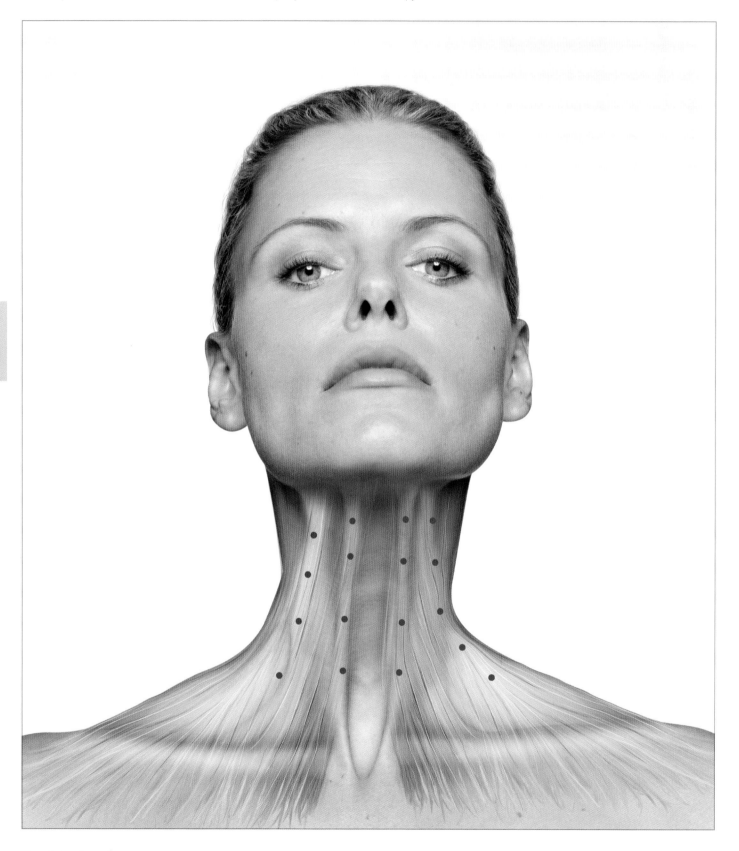

Treatment regimen
The injections are given in each cord at 2-cm intervals.

⚠ Please observe the off-label therapy warnings relating to the licensed products (cf. section 1.12, p. 8) and the relevant product inserts.

Treatment

Injection

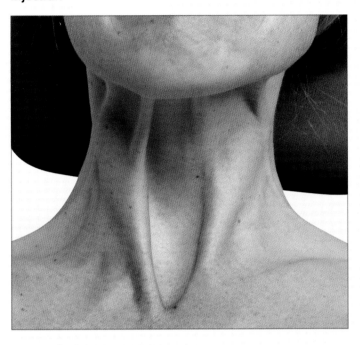

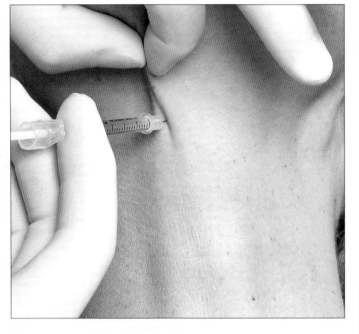

Activation
The practitioner instructs the patient to contract the muscle actively: "Pull the corners of your mouth and your lower lip hard downwards and sideways and tighten the skin of your neck."

Injection technique
Using the thumb and index finger, the therapist gently lifts the individual, tightened cords or bands.
The injections are given directly into the muscle, from top to bottom and strictly at 2-cm intervals, always ensuring that the needle is not inserted too deep.

Products and doses

Injection site	Product	Units/point	Ml solution/point
Platysma	**Xeomin**	1–2	0.025–0.05
	Botox	1–2	0.025–0.05
	Dysport	2.5–5	0.0125–0.025

Table 5.16 The authors' consensus dose recommendations for the treatment of platysmal bands. The same data apply for products with identical substance preparations.

Correction factor
Man with active expressions: Factor 2
Age / inactive expressions: Factor 0.5.

Combined treatment options
Horizontal lines can be treated with augmentation methods.

Complications / Managing complications

If the injection is too deep, BTX-A can diffuse into the underlying muscles and lead to difficulties with swallowing and speech. Therefore, injections into the laryngeal region should be avoided if at all possible.
Slight bleeding or minor hematomas may occur after the injections.

5

5.15 Primary hyperhidrosis | Eccrine sweat glands

Findings evaluation

Primary hyperhidrosis generally occurs focally, in circumscribed areas of the body. No underlying internal or external causes are present. The predilection sites are the armpits, soles of the feet, palms of the hands, forehead and neck. These regions exhibit a high density of eccrine sweat glands.

Predilection sites for primary hyperhidrosis

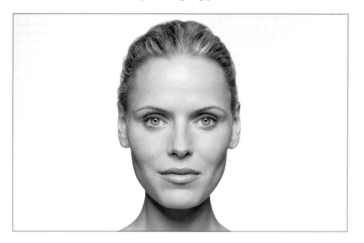
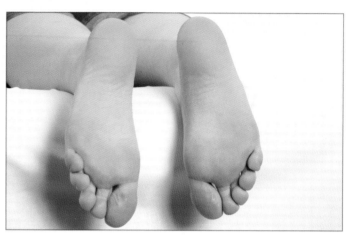
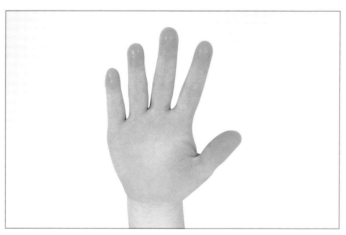
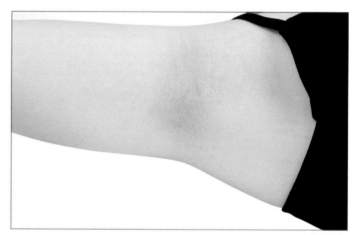

Patient selection

Treatment with botulinum toxin leads to inhibition of the sympathetic cholinergic nerve fibers and reduces or prevents sweat production. Treatment is indicated if conventional topical measures (e.g. products for external use containing aluminum chloride hexahydrate or tannic acid) fail to adequately reduce sweat production and the condition causes the patient considerable distress.

Assessing the indication

The intradermal injection of botulinum toxin A is one of the most effective methods of reducing excessive sweat production. Considerably longer durations of action are observed when treating hyperhidrosis than with cosmetic procedures: remissions have occurred only after 6 to 12 months, and as much as 18 months in some cases. The causes of this have not been fully clarified as yet.

⚠ Please observe the off-label therapy warnings relating to the licensed products (cf. section 1.12, p. 8) and the relevant product inserts.

The Minor test

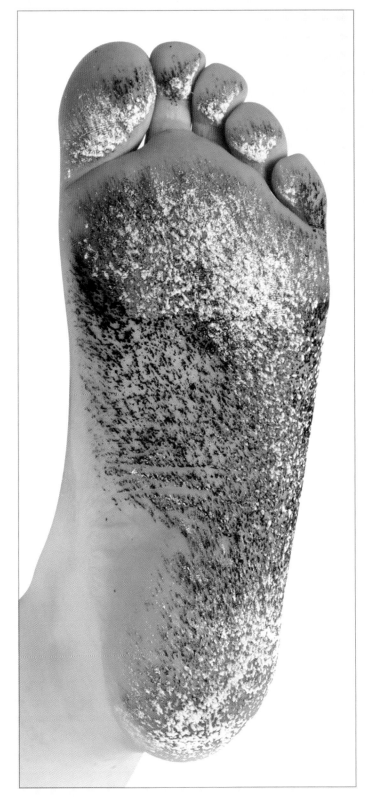

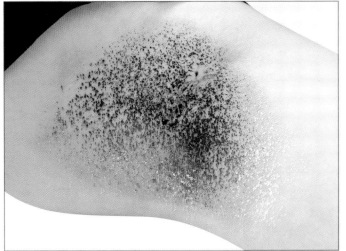

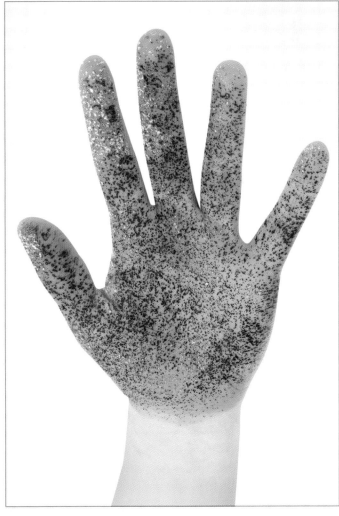

The Minor test

The affected areas are first delineated using the Minor test. The first step involves the application of Lugol's solution (iodine/potassium io-dide solution) with a swab. The second step is to dust the area with cornstarch. After 3 to 5 minutes (the waiting time varies individually), the sweat-producing skin areas become discolored, because dissol-ved polyiodide ions become deposited in the starch molecule.

Planning of treatment

Sweating is an important thermoregulatory function. In patients with axillary, palmar or plantar hyperhidrosis, the condition is independent of thermoregulation. The Minor test described above is recommended for the hands and feet, as the distribution of hyperhidrotic areas can be vary variable.

Treatment regimen

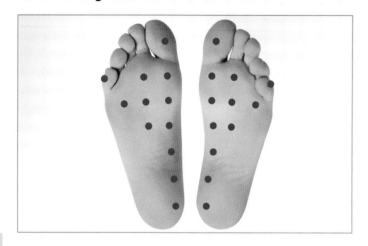

Treatment regimen for the foot
The injections are given at intervals of about 2 cm. Guide lines may be drawn to help identify the correct locations. Between 10 to 50 injection sites will be needed on the foot (examples of injection sites are shown here – there is no set injection scheme).

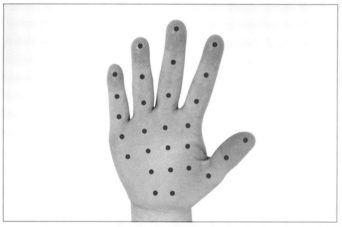

Treatment regimen for the hand
The injections are given at intervals of about 2 cm. Guide lines may be drawn to help identify the correct locations. Between 10 to 30 injection sites will be needed on the hands (examples of injection sites are shown here – there is no set injection scheme).

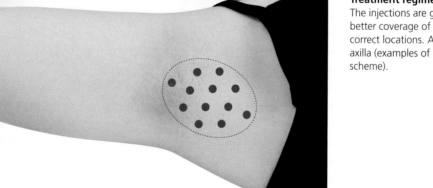

Treatment regimen for the axilla
The injections are given at intervals of about 2 cm, but may be staggered for better coverage of the area. Guidelines may be drawn to help identify the correct locations. About 10 or more injection sites will be needed in the axilla (examples of injection sites are shown here – there is no set injection scheme).

Practical tip

Pay particular attention to the lateral areas on the foot, as increased sweat production can also occur here. The needles used for the axillary, palmar or plantar injections should be about 10–20 mm in length. In the armpit, the region of highest sweat production is usually identical to the area of hair growth. This area can be relatively large in men.

⚠ Please observe the off-label therapy warnings relating to the licensed products (cf. section 1.12, p. 8) and the relevant product inserts.

Treatment

Injection

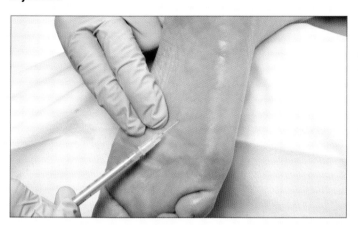

Injection technique for the foot
By preference, the injections are given intradermally, but sometimes also subcutaneously. The lateral side of the foot should also be treated if the Minor test is positive.
Caution: Take care in the medial region of the foot, as paresis may occur here due to possible diffusion of the toxin.

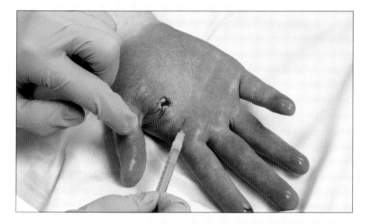

Injection technique for the hand
By preference, the injections are given intradermally, but sometimes also subcutaneously.
Caution: Take care in the thenar and hypothenar region, as muscle weakness ranging up to paresis may occur here due to possible diffusion of the toxin, making grasping difficult.

5

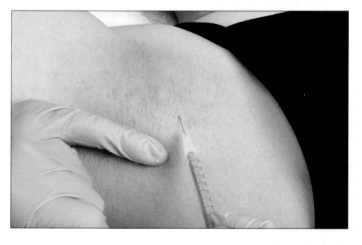

Injection technique for the axilla
By convention, the injections are given intradermally, but increasingly also subcutaneously.
Caution: Injection into the axilla is almost free of complications, but local hematomas may develop.

Products and doses

Injection site	Product	Units/point	Ml solution/point
Foot/hand/axilla	**Xeomin**	2.5–5	0.0625–0.125
	Botox	2.5–5	0.0625–0.125
	Dysport	10–20	0.05–0.1

Table 5.17 The authors' consensus dose recommendations for the treatment of primary hyperhidrosis. The same data apply for products with identical substance preparations.

 Complications / Managing complications

The injection is usually very painful in the hands and feet, so that anesthetic measures (e.g. conduction anesthesia) may be necessary.

6 Case histories

6 Case histories

Horizontal forehead lines – Case 1

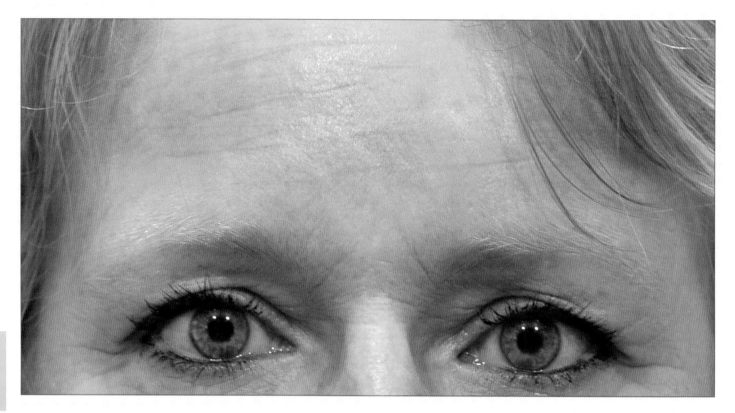

Baseline finding: very pronounced horizontal forehead lines at rest.

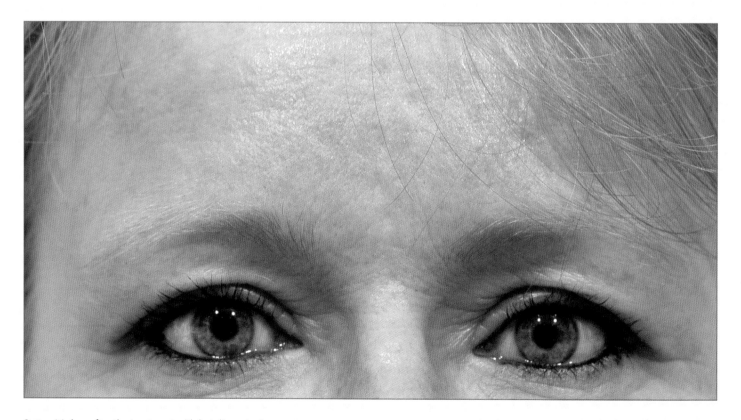

Status 14 days after the treatment with botulinum toxin.

Horizontal forehead lines – Case 2

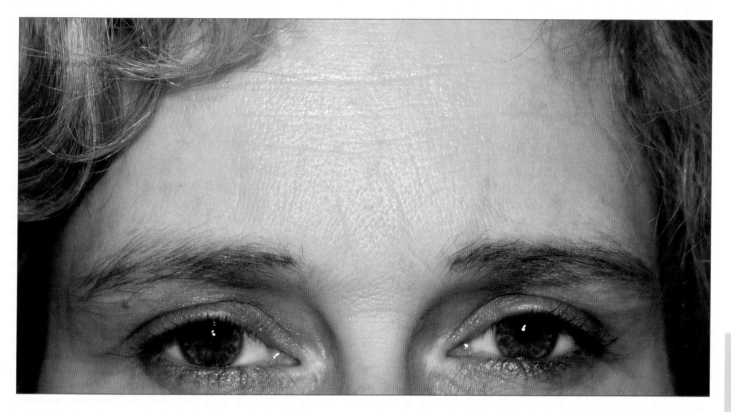

Baseline finding: very pronounced horizontal forehead lines at rest.

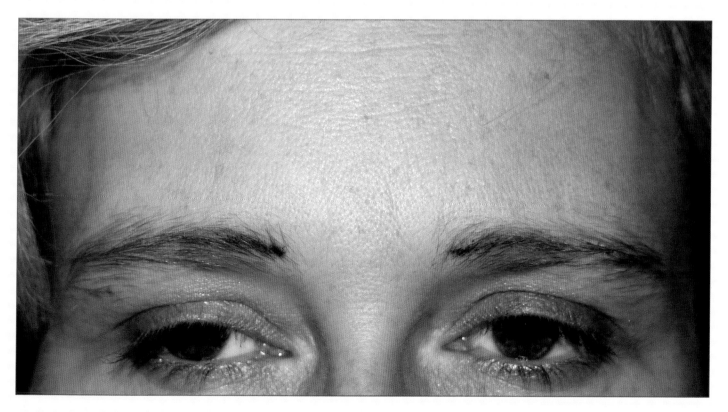

Status 14 days after the treatment with botulinum toxin.

Glabella (frown line) – Case 1

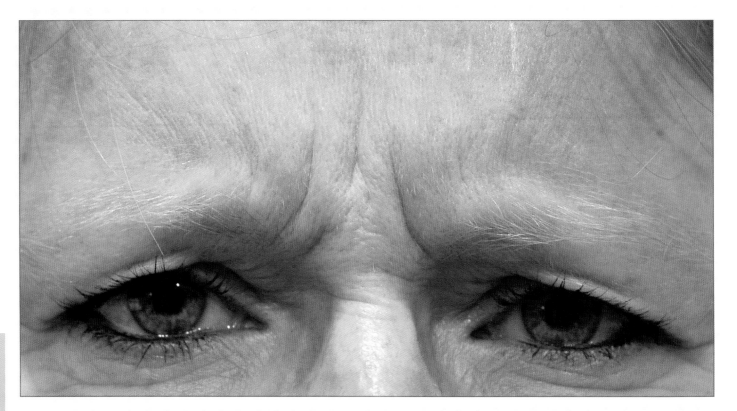

Baseline finding: very pronounced frown line on voluntary contraction.

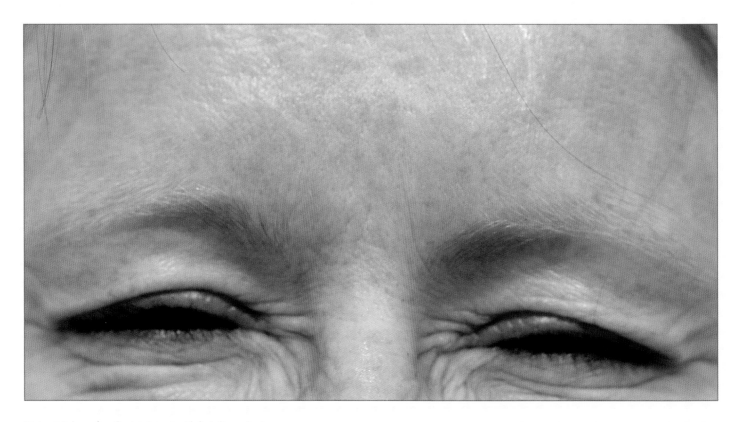

Status 14 days after the treatment with botulinum toxin.

Glabella (frown line) – Case 2

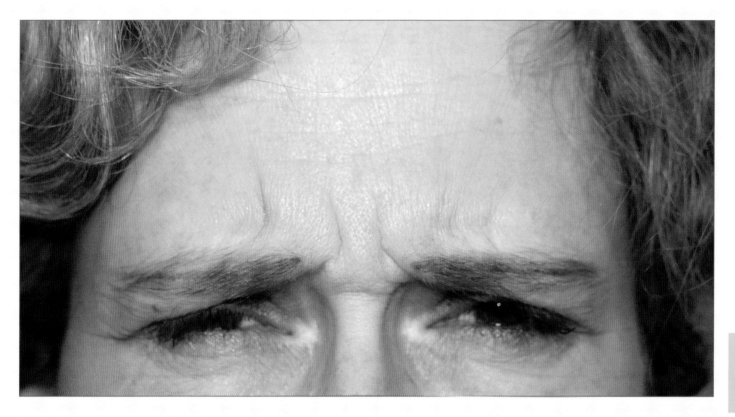

Baseline finding: very pronounced frown line on voluntary contraction.

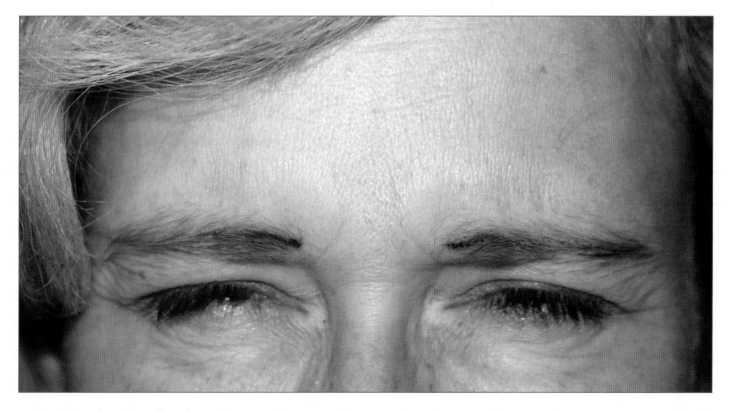

Status 14 days after the treatment with botulinum toxin.

Chemical brow lift – Case 1

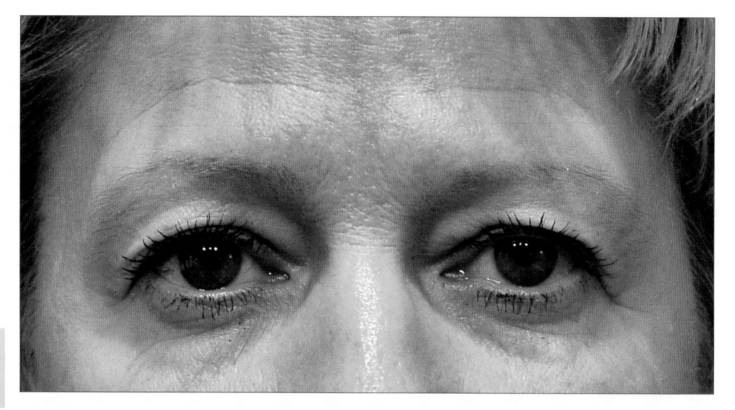

Baseline finding: slightly asymmetric, drooping brows and apparent skin excess of the upper lids produce a tired, weary look.

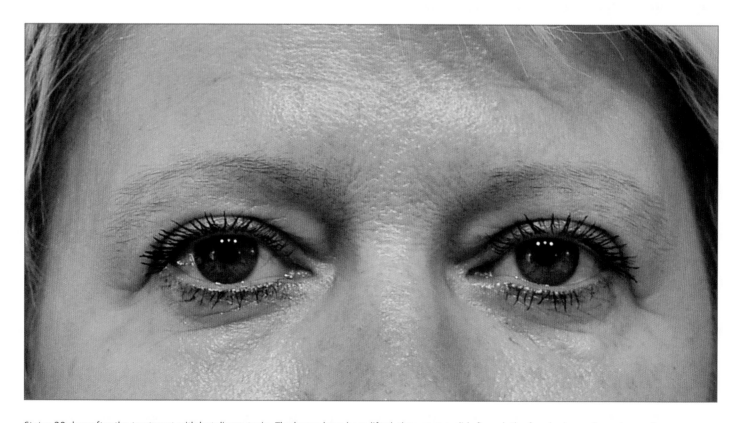

Status 20 days after the treatment with botulinum toxin. The brows have been lifted, the upper eyelids firmed; the face looks awake and receptive.

6

Chemical brow lift – Case 2

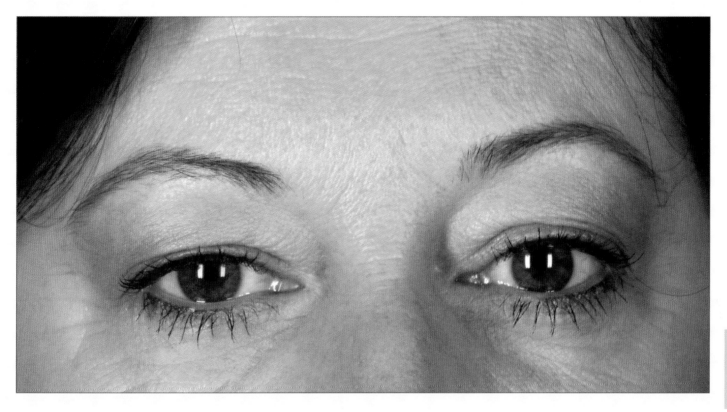

Baseline finding: the eyebrow arch has become flattened, the eyebrow height is asymmetric.

6

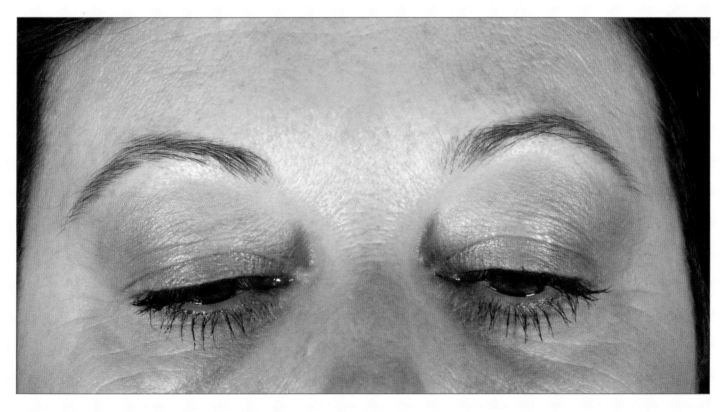

Status 14 days after the treatment with botulinum toxin: the brows have been lifted, the eyebrow arch is very pronounced.

Lateral canthal lines – Case 1

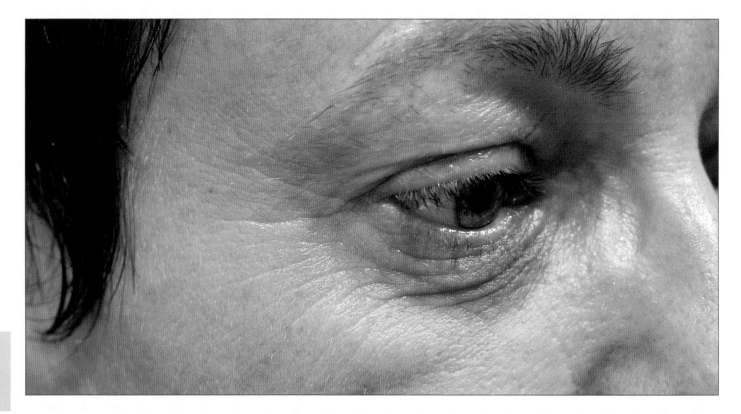

Baseline finding right: clearly visible, radial lines run from the lateral edge of the eyelid at rest.

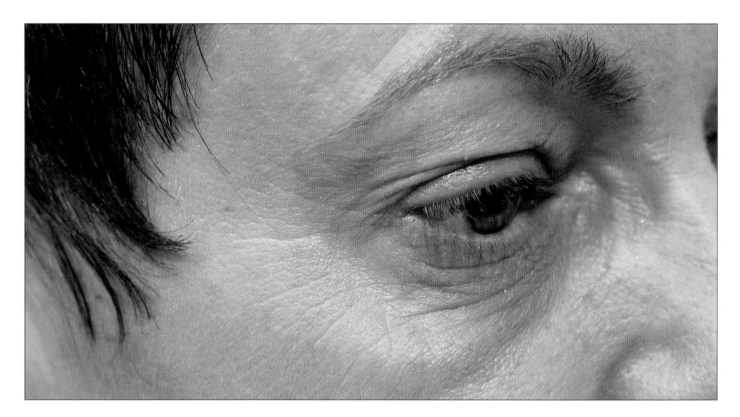

There has been a marked reduction of the lines 18 days after the treatment with botulinum toxin.

6

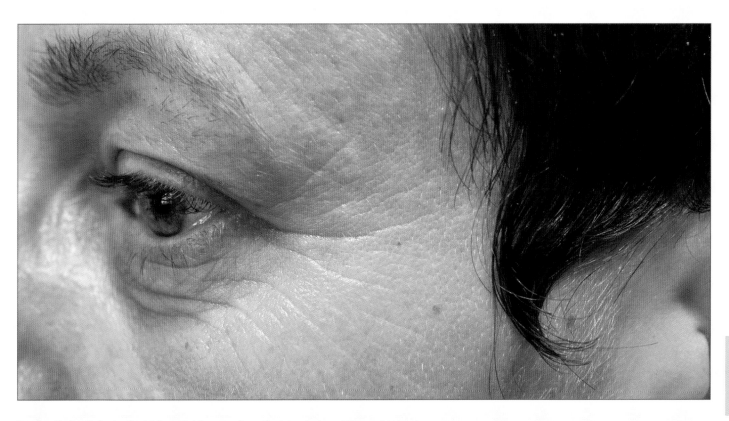

Baseline finding left: clearly visible, radial lines run from the lateral edge of the eyelid at rest.

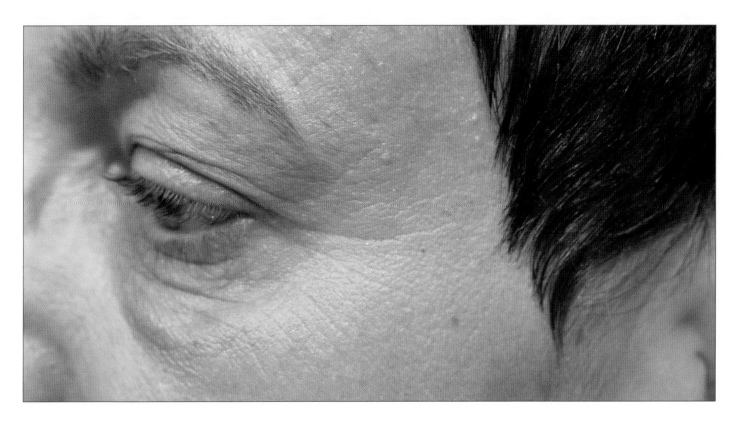

There has been a marked reduction of the lines 18 days after the treatment with botulinum toxin.

Lateral canthal lines – Case 2

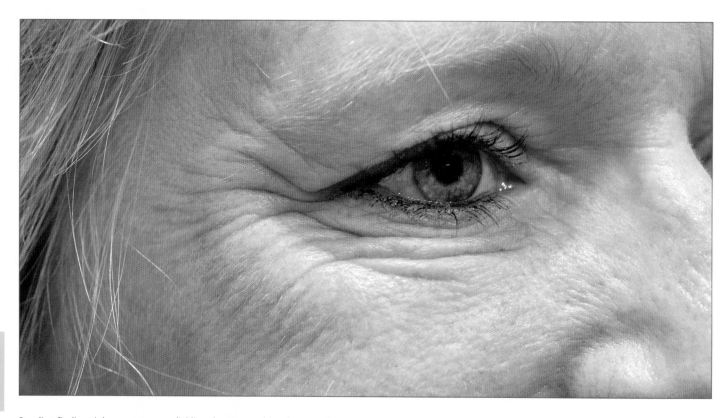

Baseline finding right: numerous radial lines become visible when the patient laughs.

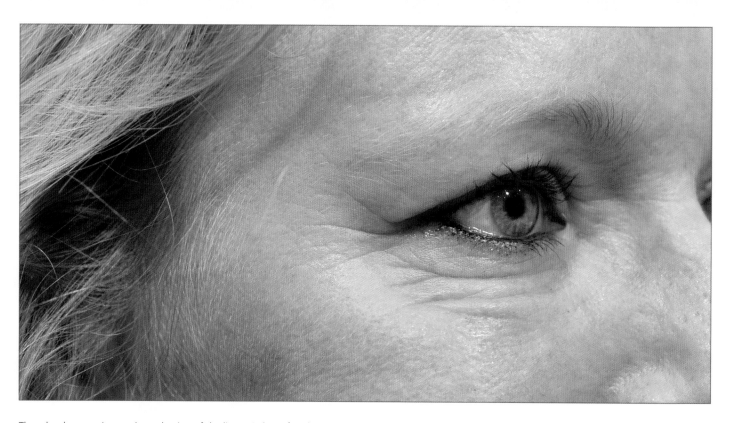

There has been an impressive reduction of the lines 13 days after the treatment with botulinum toxin.

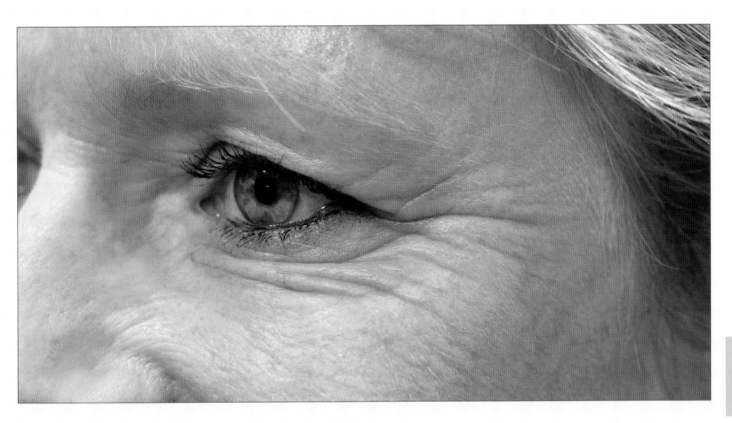

Baseline finding left: numerous radial lines become visible when the patient laughs.

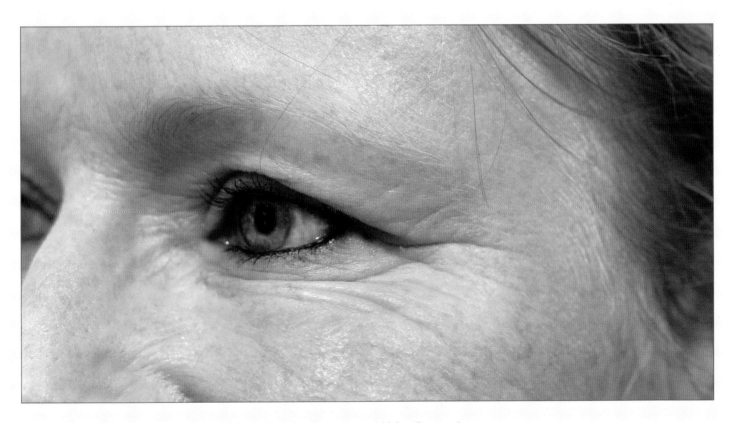

There has been an impressive reduction of the lines 13 days after the treatment with botulinum toxin.

6

Fine skin creases on the lower eyelid

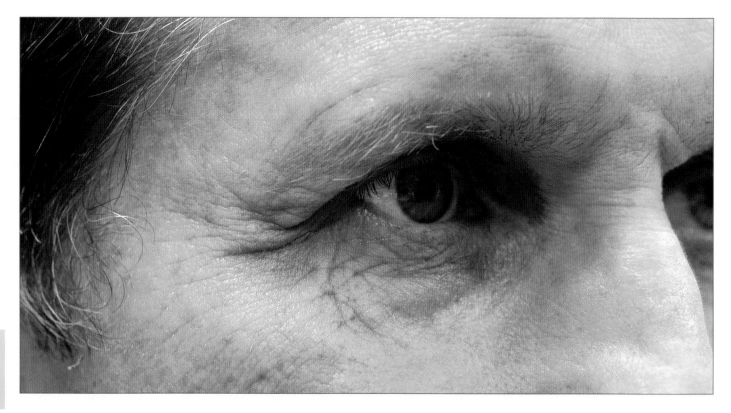

Baseline finding right: clearly visible, fine wrinkling of the periorbital skin at rest.

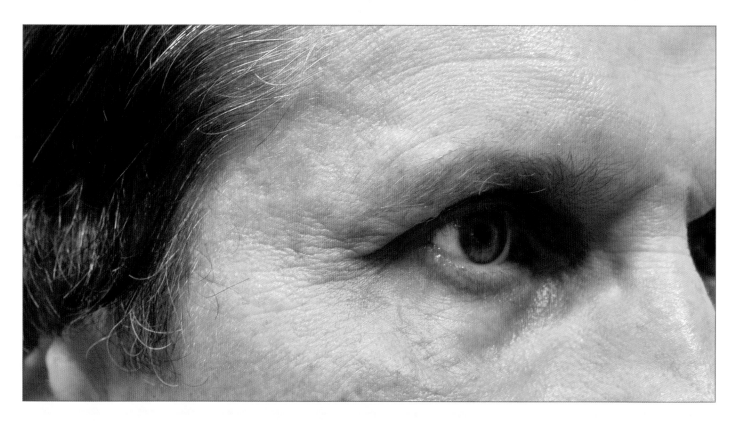

Marked smoothing of the skin and reduction of the lines can be seen 16 days after the treatment with botulinum toxin.

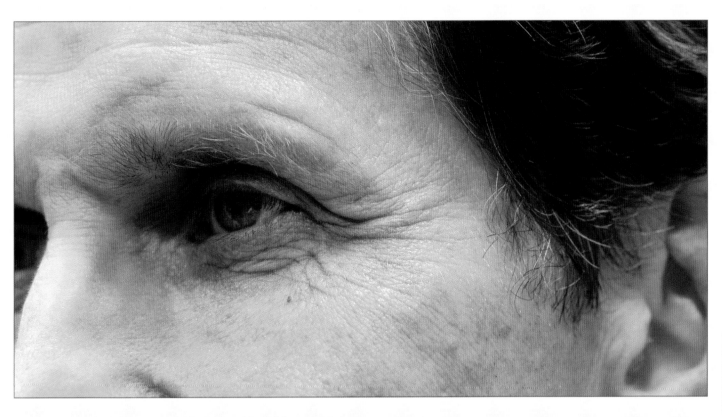

Baseline finding left: there is clearly visible, fine wrinkling of the periorbital skin at rest.

6

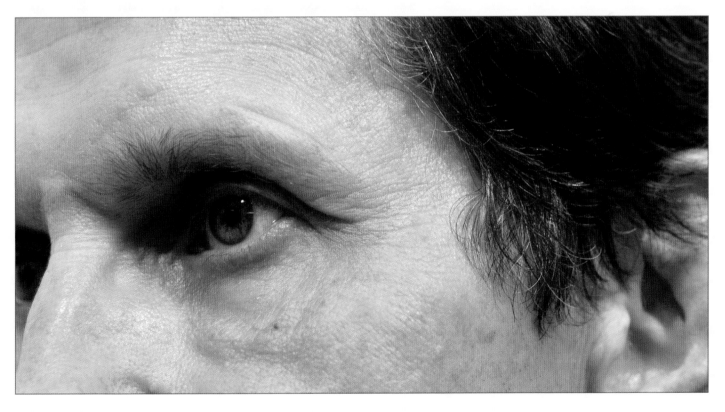

Marked smoothing of the skin and reduction of the lines can be seen 16 days after the treatment with botulinum toxin.

Bunny lines – Case 1

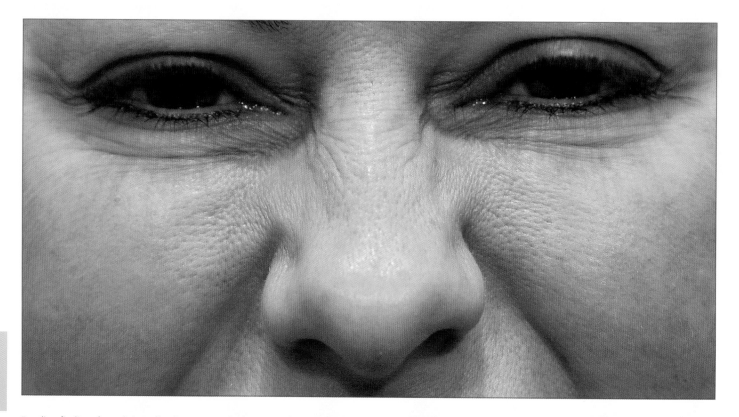

Baseline finding, frontal view: fine lines appear in the upper third of the nose when the patient laughs.

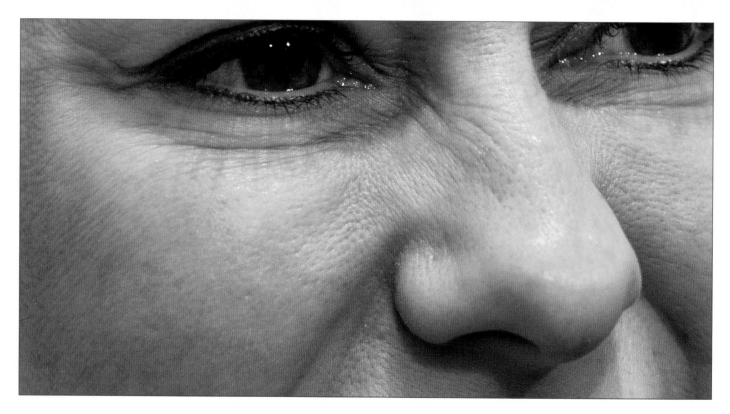

Baseline finding right: clearly visible lines in the lateral upper third of the nose.

6

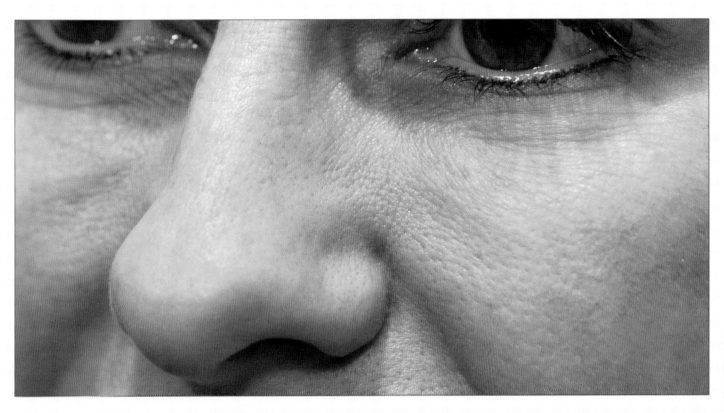

Right: 14 days after the treatment with botulinum toxin, lines are no longer visible when the patient laughs.

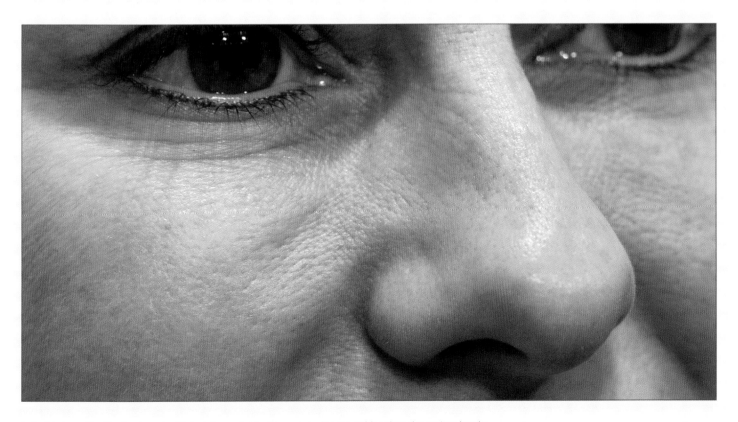

Left: 14 days after the treatment with botulinum toxin, lines are no longer visible when the patient laughs.

Bunny lines – Case 2

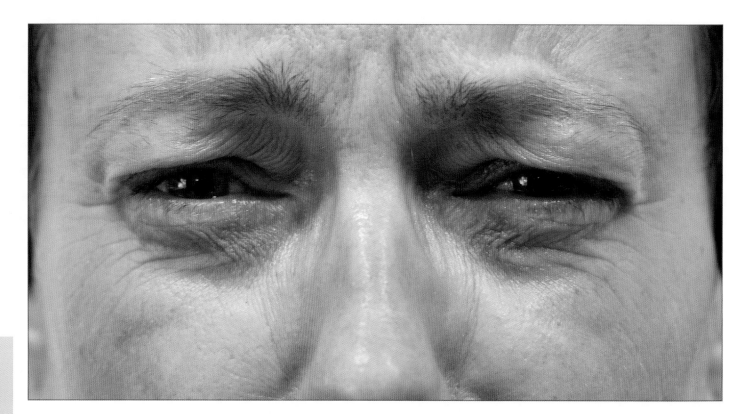

Baseline finding, frontal view: the baseline assessment shows a glabellar line, which can be produced dynamically.

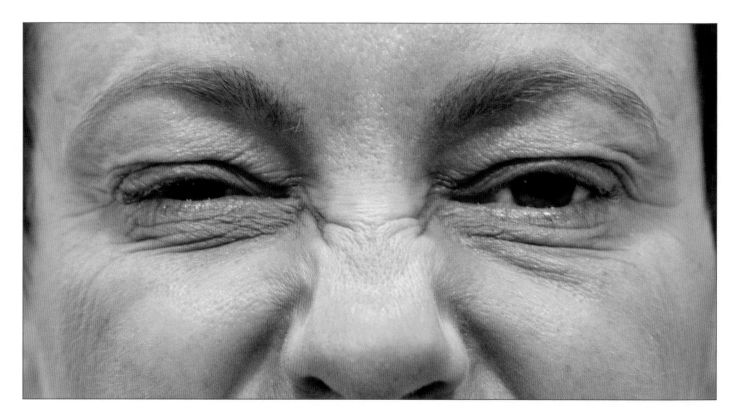

Eighteen days after the treatment with botulinum toxin, the glabellar line can no longer be actively produced. However, fine nasal lines are now visible in the middle and upper third of the nose due to compensatory activation of the nasalis muscle.

6

Gummy smile

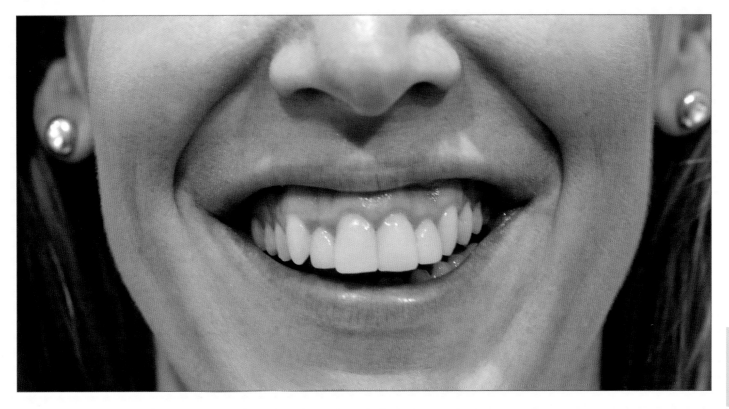

Baseline finding: a disproportionate amount of gum is exposed when the patient smiles.

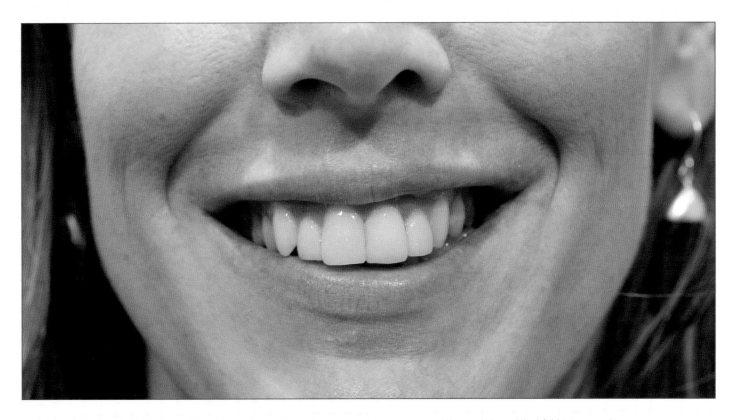

Seventeen days after the treatment with botulinum toxin, the smile looks more harmonious and the medial nasolabial fold is improved.

6

Lines around the upper and lower lip

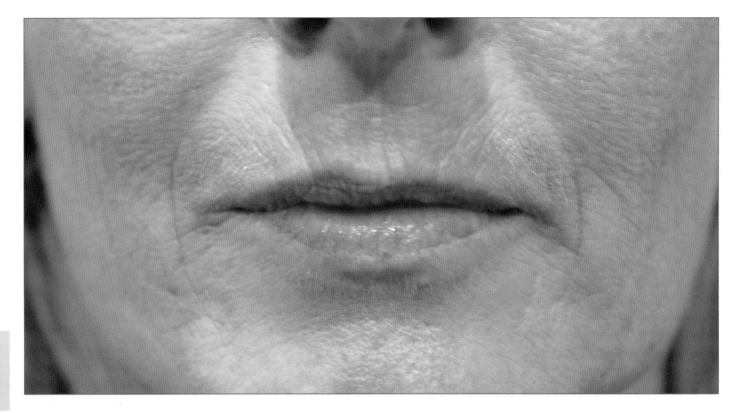

Baseline finding: at rest, marked, radial lines can be seen around the mouth, particularly in the upper lip.

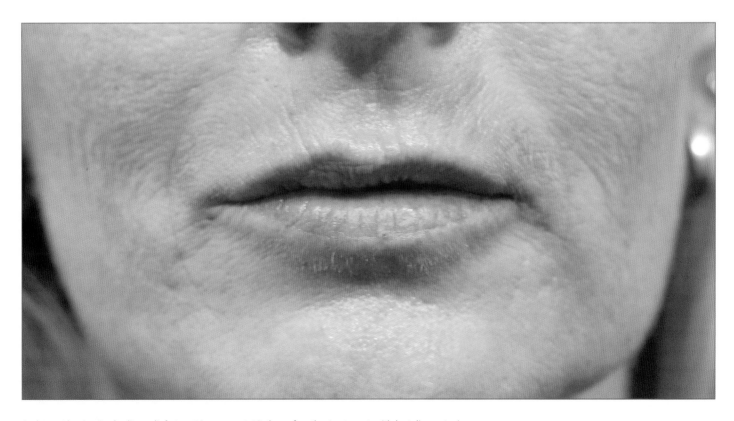

A clear reduction in the line relief at rest is apparent 13 days after the treatment with botulinum toxin.

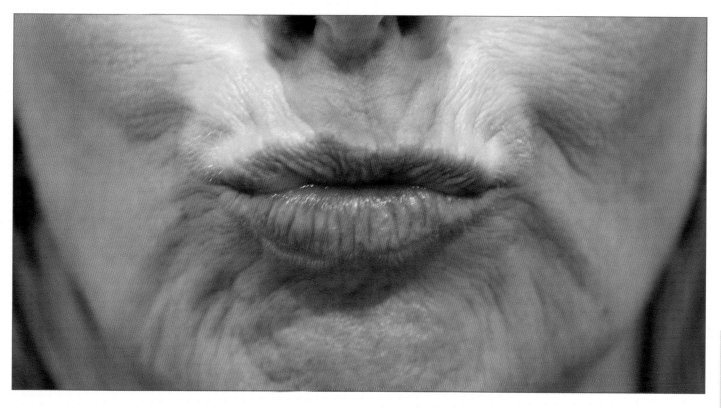

Baseline finding: active contraction of the orbicularis oris muscle makes the lines even more pronounced.

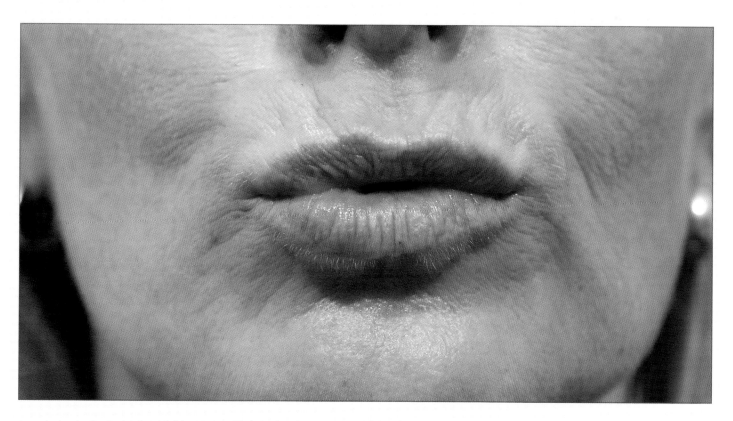

A marked reduction in the line relief is apparent 13 days after the treatment with botulinum toxin.

Marionette lines – Case 1

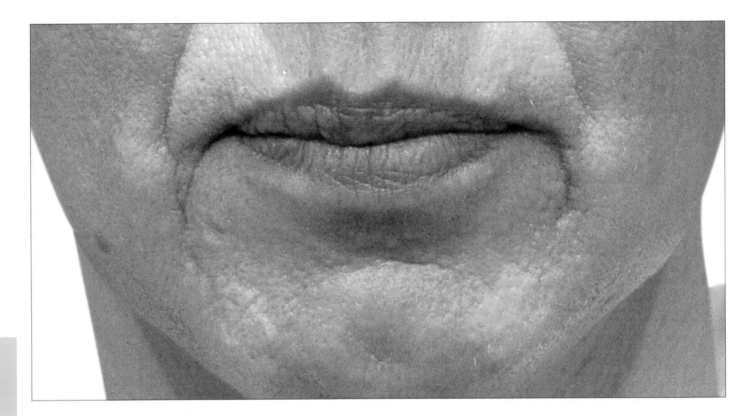

Baseline status: marionette lines are apparent on both sides of the mouth at rest.

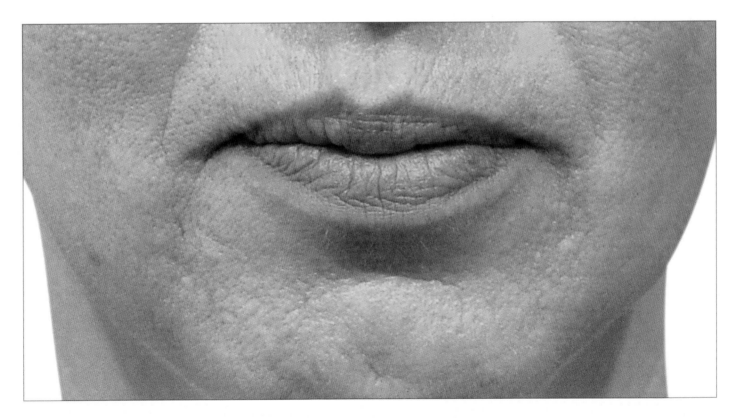

The lines have become almost invisible 14 days after the treatment with botulinum toxin.

Cobblestone chin – Case 1

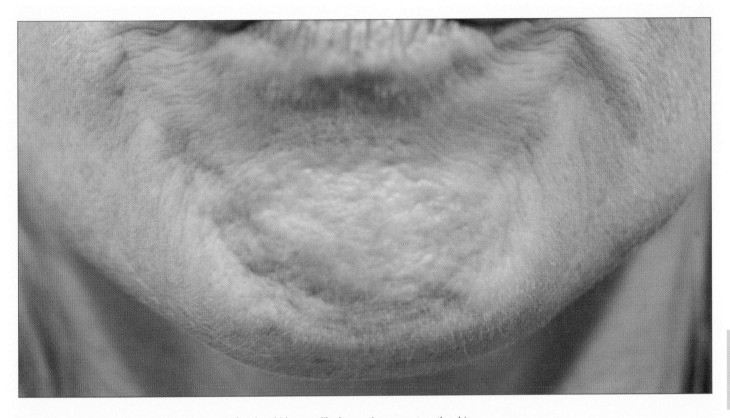

Baseline status: an irregularly structured skin relief with cobblestone-like bumps is apparent on the chin.

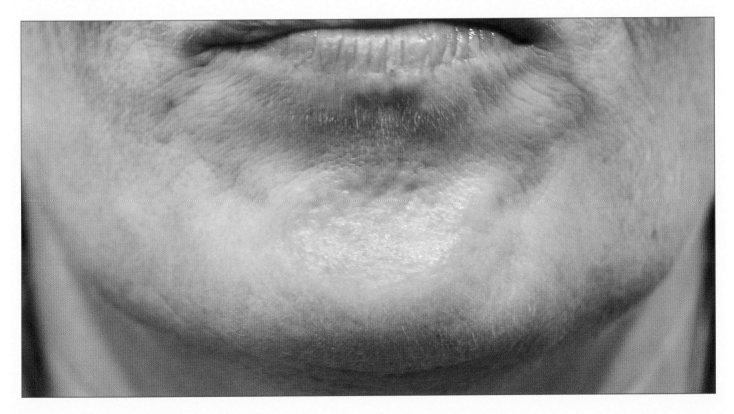

Thirteen days after a treatment with botulinum toxin, the skin looks almost completely smooth.

6

Cobblestone chin – Case 2

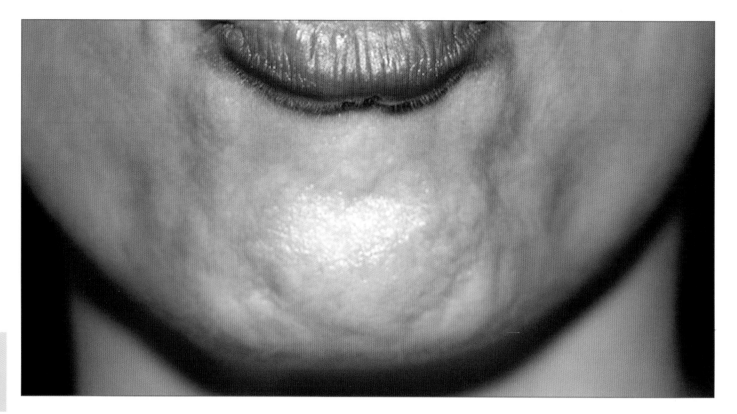

Baseline status: an irregularly structured skin relief with cobblestone-like bumps is apparent on the chin.

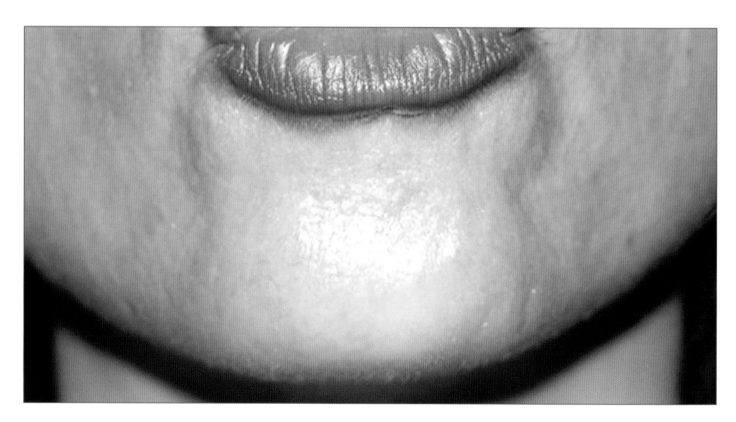

Marked smoothing is apparent 14 days after a treatment with botulinum toxin.

6

Platysmal bands – Case 1

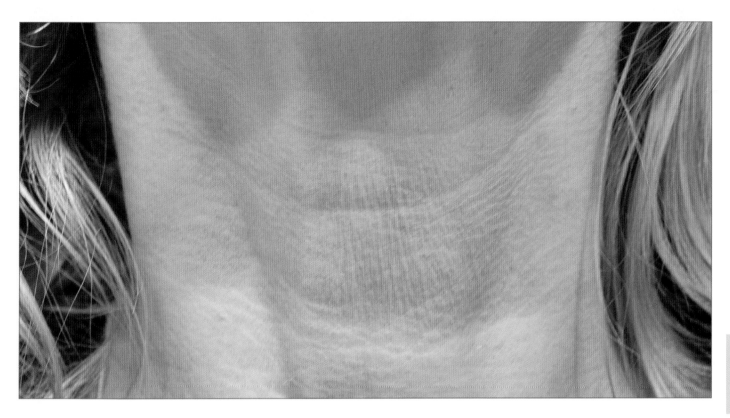

Baseline status: very thin, fine, vertical lines can be seen, particularly in the ventral region.

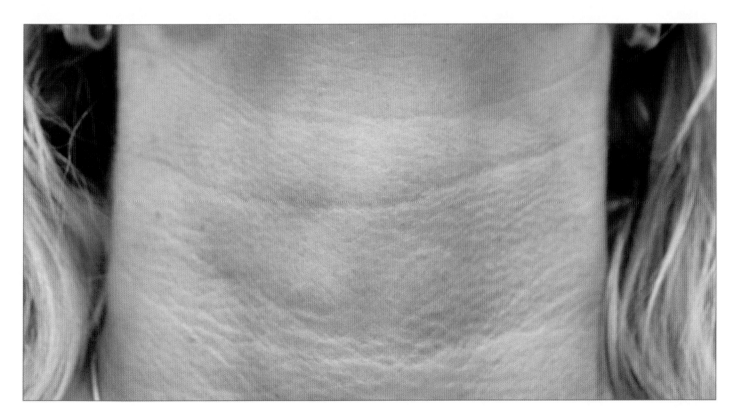

Fourteen days after a treatment with botulinum toxin, there has been impressive smoothing of the fine platysmal bands. The horizontal lines are not improved.

Platysmal bands – Case 2

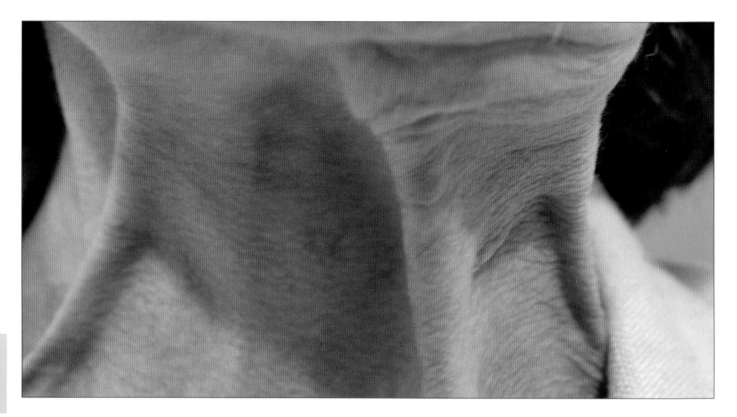

Baseline status: very pronounced bands can be seen in the lateral and ventral regions.

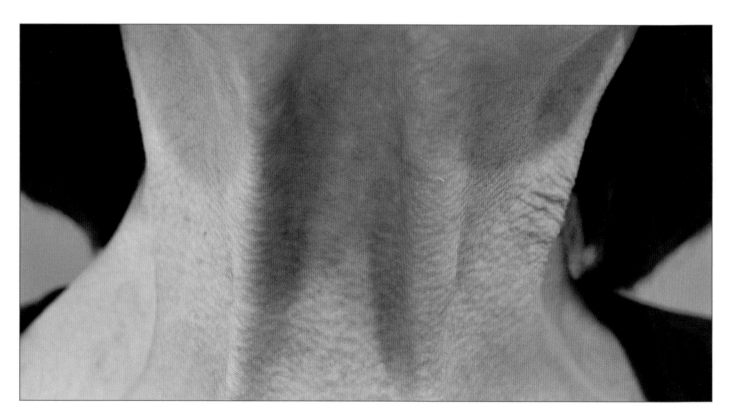

Fourteen days after a treatment with botulinum toxin, the lateral bands have almost completely disappeared. The bands in the ventral region have become less pronounced in this patient with excess and lax neck skin.

Top third of the face – Case 1

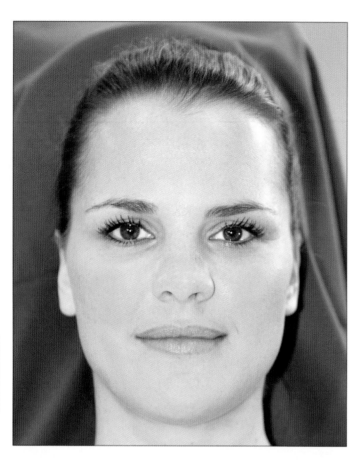

Baseline status at rest.

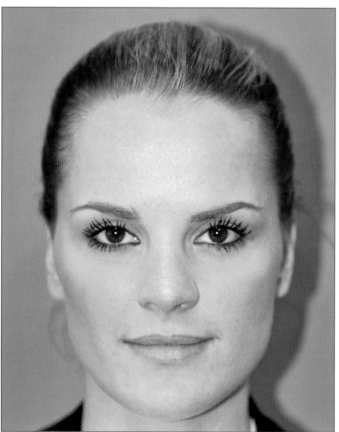

One month after a treatment with botulinum toxin, notable brow lift and general improvement of the patient's expression and skin appearance.

Baseline status

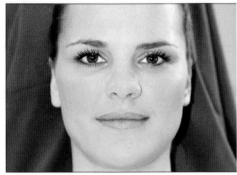 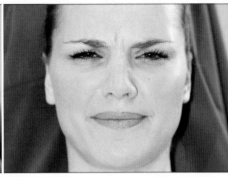 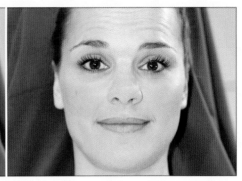

At rest.   At active depression.   At active elevation.

One week after treatment

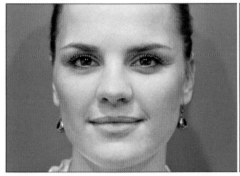 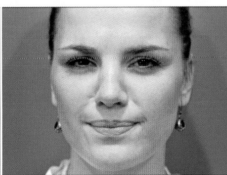 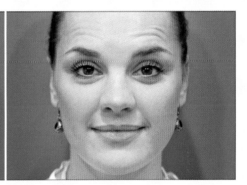

At rest.   At active depression.   At active elevation.

6

One month after treatment

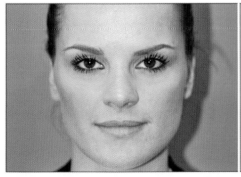 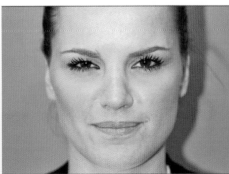 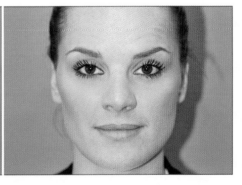

At rest.   At active depression.   At active elevation.

Video: "Top third of the face – case 1"
http://www.kvm-tv.de/BTX/btx014.mp4

Top third of the face – Case 2

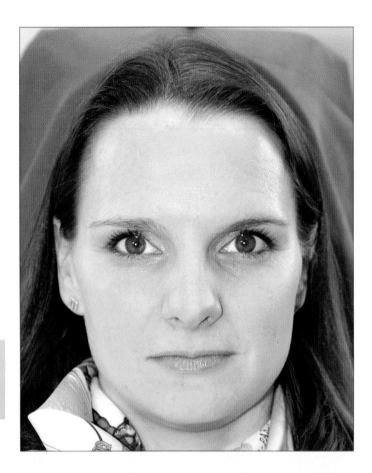

Baseline status at rest.

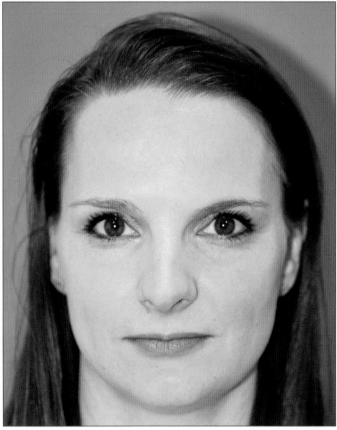

One month after a treatment with botulinum toxin, clearly visible, the patient's look is more awake and relaxed, and the horizontal lines on her forehead are smoothed.

6

Baseline status

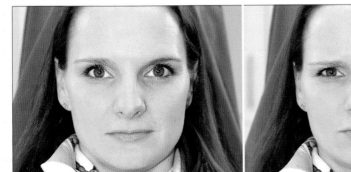 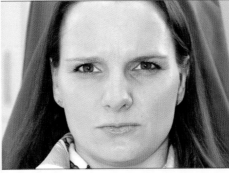 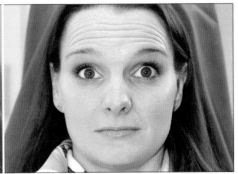

At rest.　　　　　　　　　At active depression.　　　　　　　At active elevation.

One week after treatment

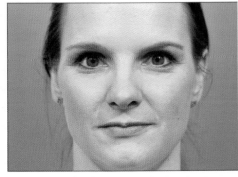 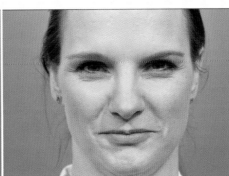 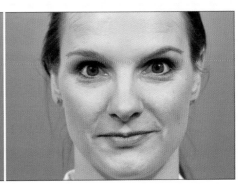

At rest.　　　　　　　　　At active depression.　　　　　　　At active elevation.

One month after treatment

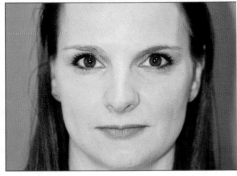 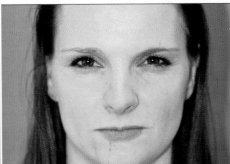 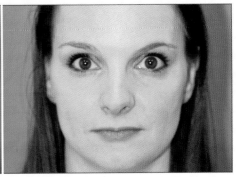

At rest.　　　　　　　　　At active depression.　　　　　　　At active elevation.

 Video: "Top third of the face – case 2"
http://www.kvm-tv.de/BTX/btx015.mp4

6

Top third of the face – Case 3

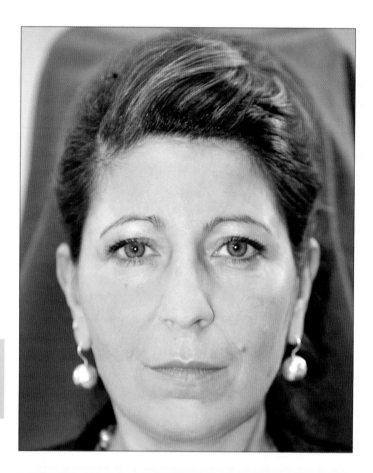

Baseline status at rest.

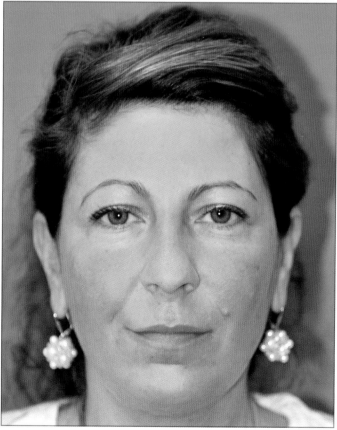

One month after a treatment with botulinum toxin, marked smoothing of the skin together with a natural brow lift.

6

Baseline status

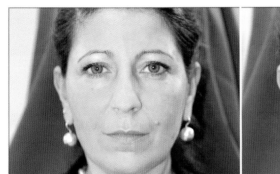 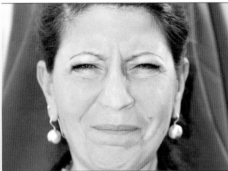 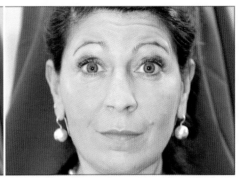

At rest.   At active depression.   At active elevation.

One week after treatment

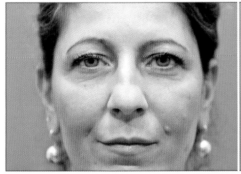 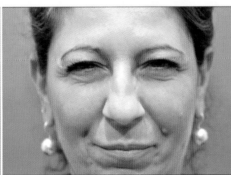 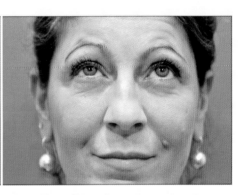

At rest.   At active depression.   At active elevation.

One month after treatment

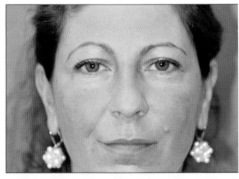 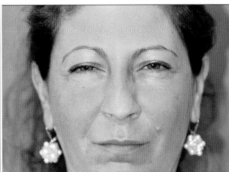 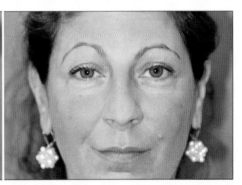

At rest.   At active depression.   At active elevation.

 Video: "Top third of the face – case 3"
http://www.kvm-tv.de/BTX/btx016.mp4

Top third of the face – Case 4

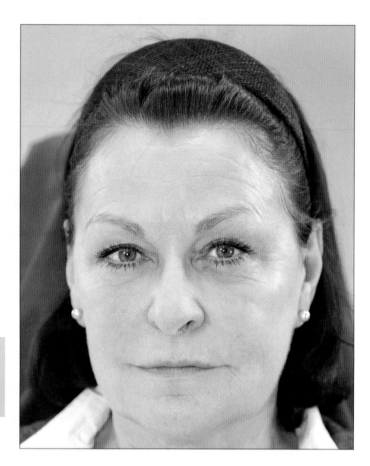

Baseline status at rest.

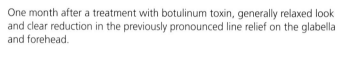

One month after a treatment with botulinum toxin, generally relaxed look and clear reduction in the previously pronounced line relief on the glabella and forehead.

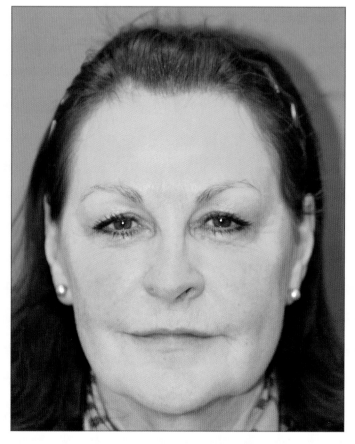

6

Baseline status

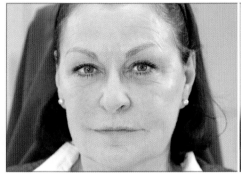 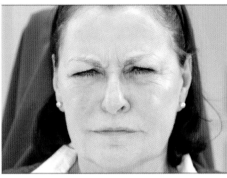 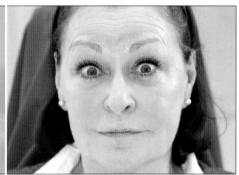

At rest.   At active depression.   At active elevation.

One week after treatment

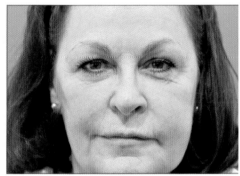 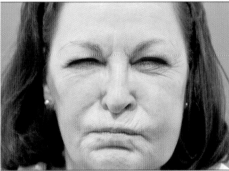 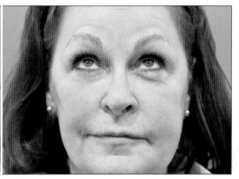

At rest.   At active depression.   At active elevation.

6

One month after treatment

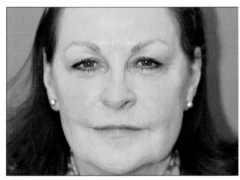 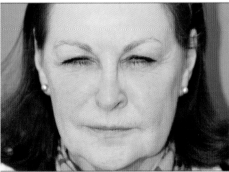 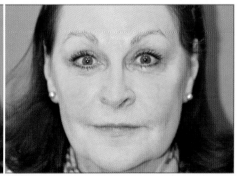

At rest.   At active depression.   At active elevation.

 Video: "Top third of the face – case 4"
http://www.kvm-tv.de/BTX/btx017.mp4

Top third of the face – Case 5

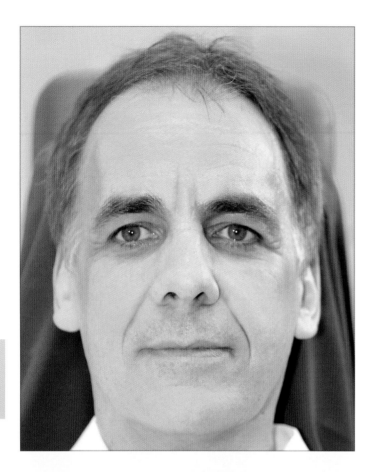

Baseline status at rest.

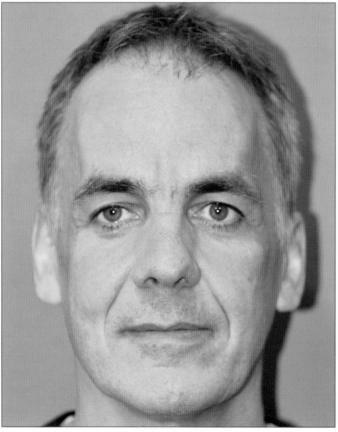

One month after a treatment with botulinum toxin: an impressive reduction in the once very pronounced line relief on the gleballa and forehead coupled with marked brow lift and a general improvement of the patient's look ("opened eyes") and skin appearance.

6

Baseline status

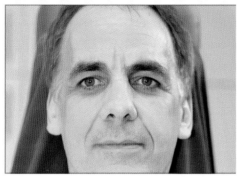 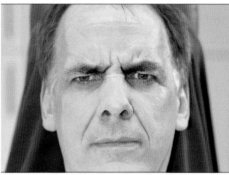 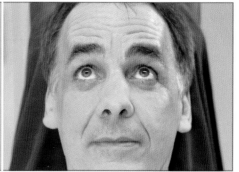

At rest.   At active depression.   At active elevation.

One week after treatment

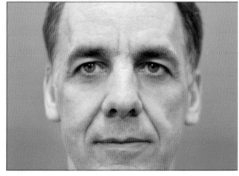 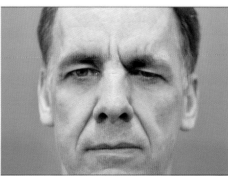 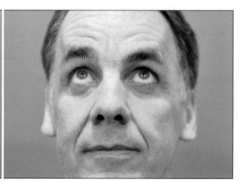

At rest.   At active depression.   At active elevation.

One month after treatment

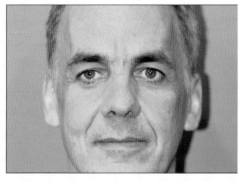 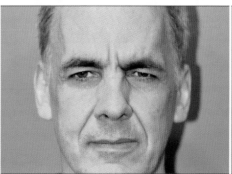 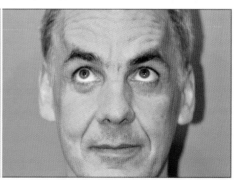

At rest.   At active depression.   At active elevation.

Video: "Top third of the face – case 5"
http://www.kvm-tv.de/BTX/btx018.mp4

7 Aids for the practitioner

Documentation Form for Aesthetic Treatments

Name of patient _____ Date of birth _____ Medical Insurance _____

Treatment with: ☐ ☐
                  Botulinum toxin   *Filler*

Products: _____

Batch numbers: _____

Units (ml): _____

Merz Scale: A B C D E F G H I J K
Value:

Date: _____

Photo today: ☐ ☐
                Yes   *No*

Treatment with: ☐ ☐
                  Botulinum toxin   *Filler*

Products: _____

Batch numbers: _____

Units (ml): _____

Merz Scale: A B C D E F G H I J K
Value:

Date: _____

Photo today: ☐ ☐
                Yes   *No*

Treatment with: ☐ ☐
                  Botulinum toxin   *Filler*

Products: _____

Batch numbers: _____

Units (ml): _____

Merz Scale: A B C D E F G H I J K
Value:

Date: _____

Photo today: ☐ ☐
                Yes   *No*

Treatment with: ☐ ☐
                  Botulinum toxin   *Filler*

Products: _____

Batch numbers: _____

Units (ml): _____

Merz Scale: A B C D E F G H I J K
Value:

Date: _____

Photo today: ☐ ☐
                Yes   *No*

Treatment with: ☐ ☐
                  Botulinum toxin   *Filler*

Products: _____

Batch numbers: _____

Units (ml): _____

Merz Scale: A B C D E F G H I J K
Value:

Date: _____

Photo today: ☐ ☐
                Yes   *No*

Treatment with: ☐ ☐
                  Botulinum toxin   *Filler*

Products: _____

Batch numbers: _____

Units (ml): _____

Merz Scale: A B C D E F G H I J K
Value:

Date: _____

Photo today: ☐ ☐
                Yes   *No*

7

Merz Aesthetic Scales

A **Brow positioning**

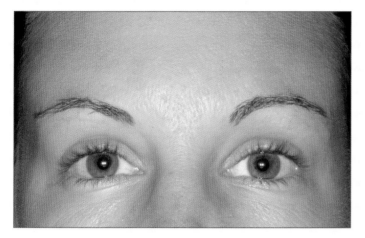

0 Youthful, refreshed look; high arch of the eyebrow

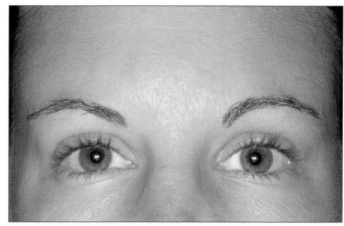

1 Medium arch of the eyebrow

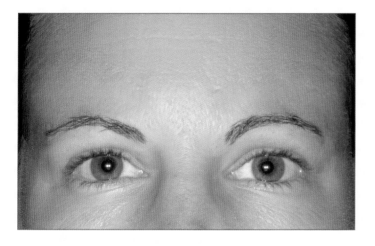

2 Slight arch of the eyebrow

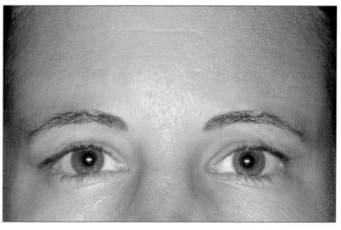

3 Flat arch of the eyebrow; visibility of folds; tired appearance

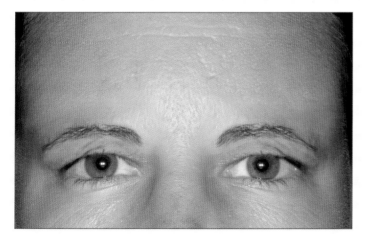

4 Flat eyebrow with barely any arch; marked visibility of folds; very tired appearance

7

B Forehead lines – at rest

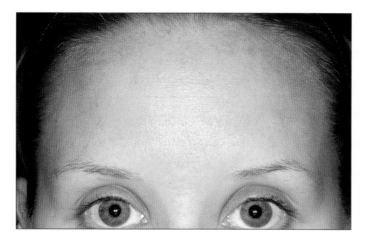

0 No lines

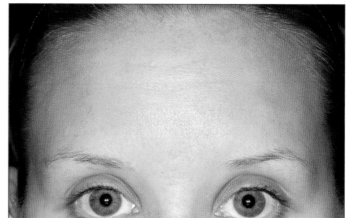

1 Mild lines

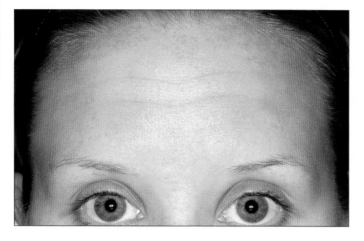

2 Moderate lines

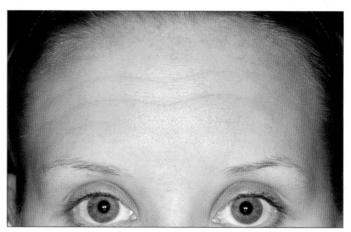

3 Severe lines

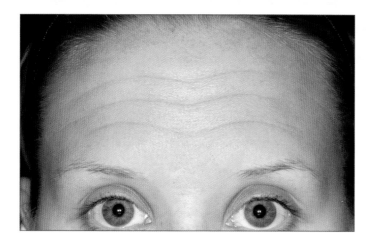

4 Very severe lines

C Forehead lines – dynamic

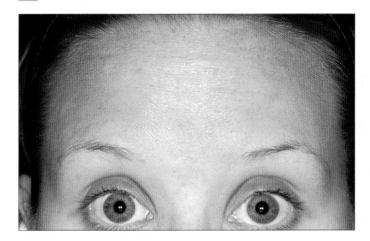

0 No lines

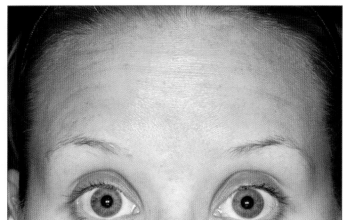

1 Mild lines

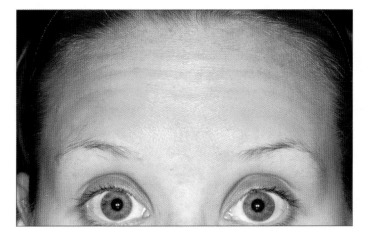

2 Moderate lines

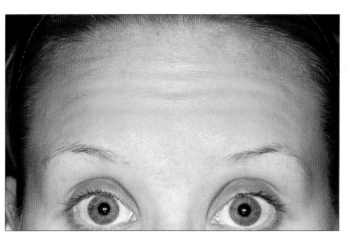

3 Severe lines

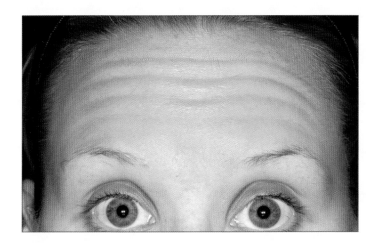

4 Very severe lines

7

D Glabellar lines – at rest

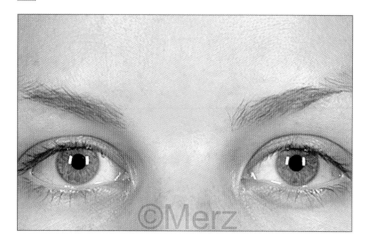

0 No glabellar lines

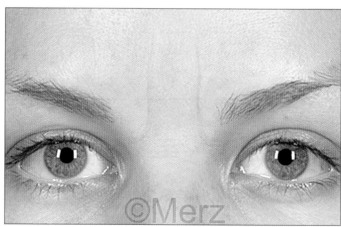

1 Mild glabellar lines

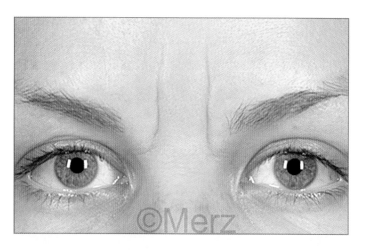

2 Moderate glabellar lines

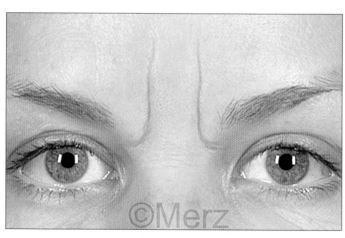

3 Severe glabellar lines

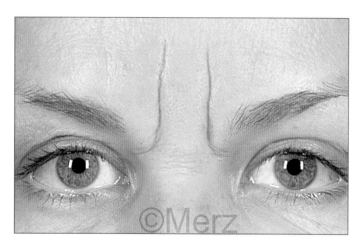

4 Very severe glabellar lines

7

E **Glabellar lines – dynamic**

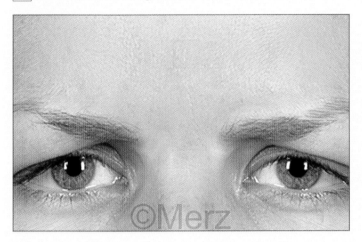

0 No lines

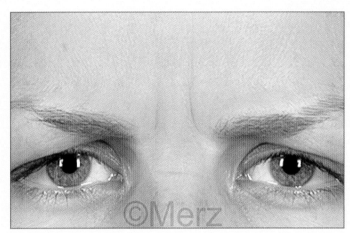

1 Mild glabellar lines

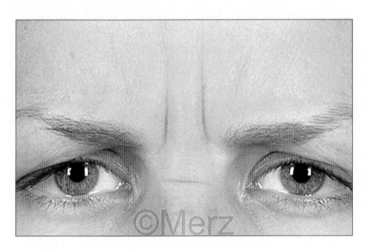

2 Moderate glabellar lines

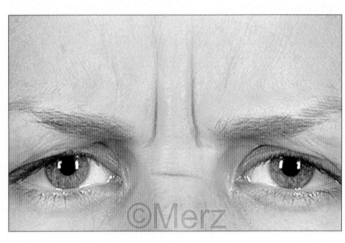

3 Severe glabellar lines

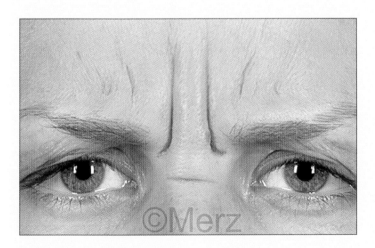

4 Very severe glabellar lines

7

F **Lateral canthal lines – at rest**

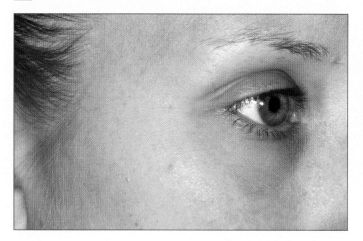

0 No lines

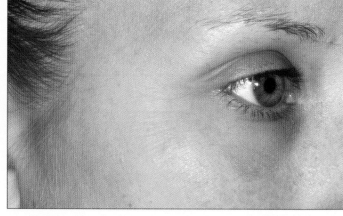

1 Mild lines

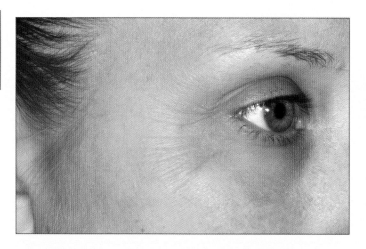

2 Moderate lines

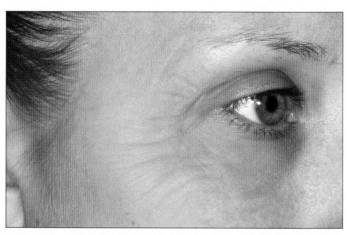

3 Severe lines

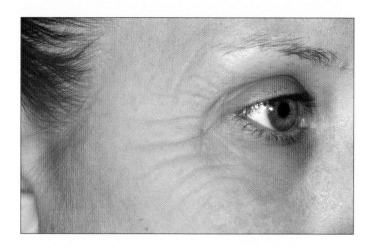

4 Very severe lines

G **Lateral canthal lines – dynamic**

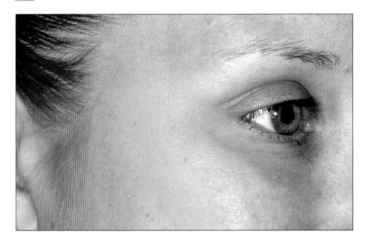

0 No lines

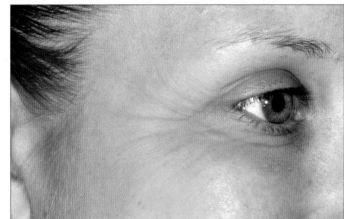

1 Mild lines

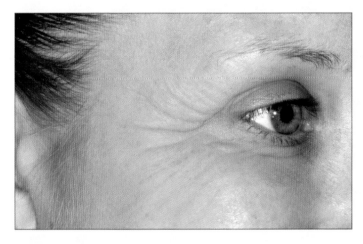

2 Moderate lines

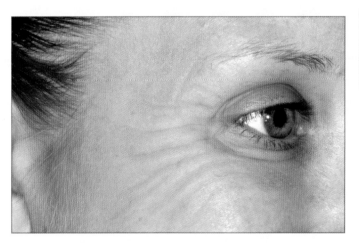

3 Severe lines

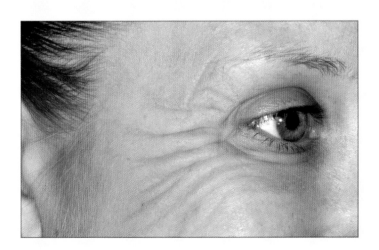

4 Very severe lines

7

H Lip wrinkles – at rest

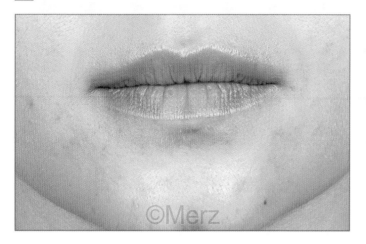

0 No wrinkles

1 Mild wrinkles

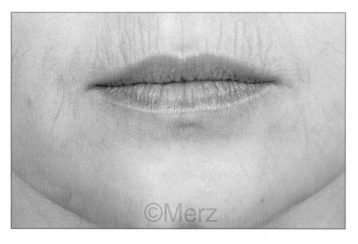

2 Moderate wrinkles

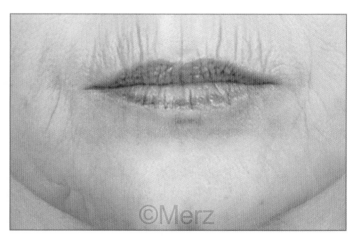

3 Severe wrinkles

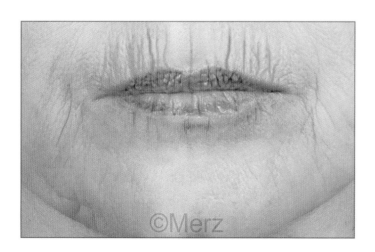

4 Very severe wrinkles

I Lip wrinkles – dynamic

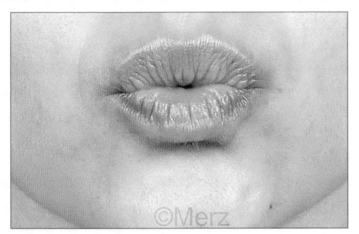

0 No wrinkles

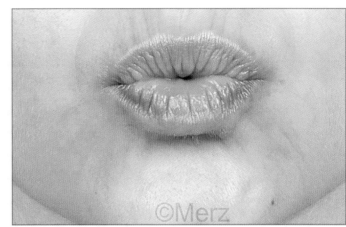

1 Mild wrinkles

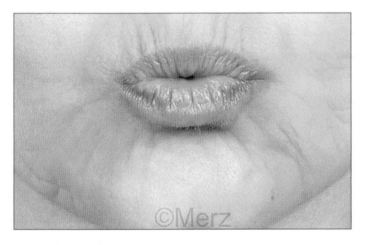

2 Moderate wrinkles

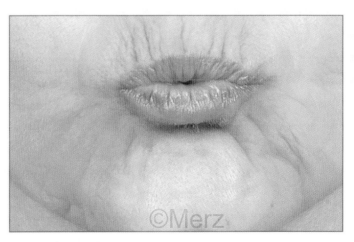

3 Severe wrinkles

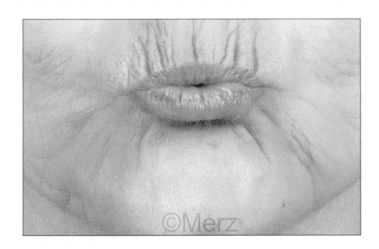

4 Very severe wrinkles

7

J **Marionette lines**

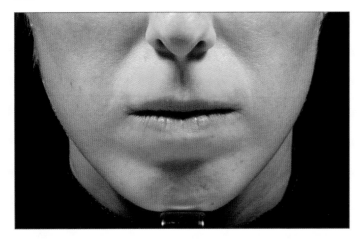

0 No lines

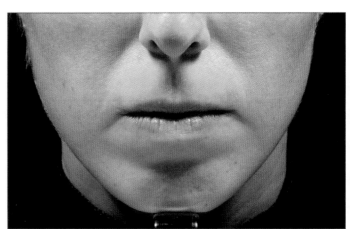

1 Mild lines

2 Moderate lines; clearly visible at rest, but not when skin is stretched

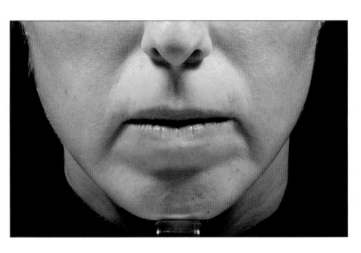

3 Severe lines, conspicuous facial feature

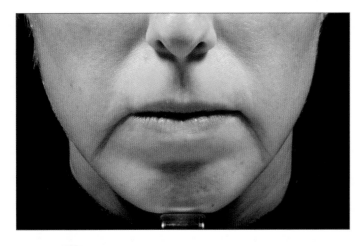

4 Very severe lines, appearance is adversely affected

7

K **Neck**

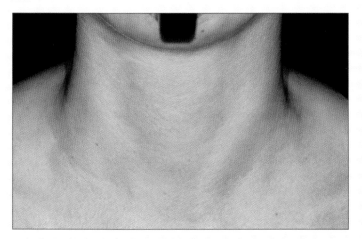

0 No visible horizontal lines or folds

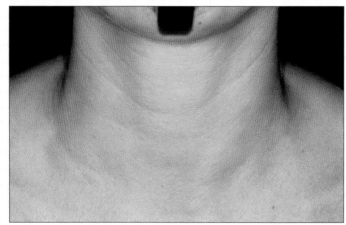

1 Mild visible horizontal lines and folds

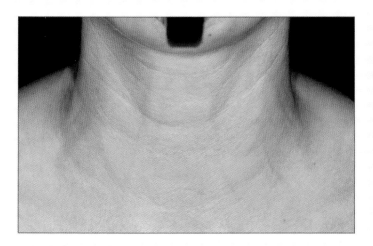

2 Moderate horizontal lines and folds; mild skin laxity and platysmal band prominence

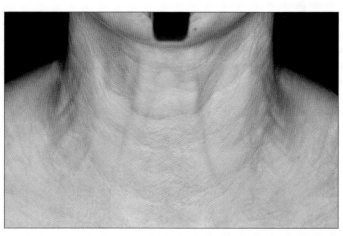

3 Severe horizontal lines and folds; moderate skin laxity and platysmal band prominence

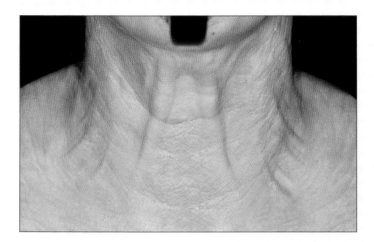

4 Very severe, deep horizontal lines and folds; severe skin laxity and platysmal band prominence

FDA Medication guides

MEDICATION GUIDE BOTOX/BOTOX Cosmetic

(Boe-tox)
(onabotulinumtoxinA)
for Injection

Read the Medication Guide that comes with **BOTOX** or **BOTOX Cosmetic** before you start using it and each time it is given to you. There may be new information. This information does not take the place of talking with your doctor about your medical condition or your treatment. You should share this information with your family members and caregivers.

What is the most important information I should know about BOTOX and BOTOX Cosmetic?

BOTOX and BOTOX Cosmetic may cause serious side effects that can be life threatening, including:
- **problems breathing or swallowing**
- **spread of toxin effects.**

These problems can happen hours, days, to weeks after an injection of BOTOX or BOTOX Cosmetic. Call your doctor or get medical help right away if you have any of these problems after treatment with BOTOX or BOTOX Cosmetic:

1. Problems swallowing, speaking, or breathing. These problems can happen hours, days, to weeks after an injection of BOTOX or BOTOX Cosmetic usually because the muscles that you use to breathe and swallow can become weak after the injection. Death can happen as a complication if you have severe problems with swallowing or breathing after treatment with **BOTOX** or **BOTOX Cosmetic**.
- People with certain breathing problems may need to use muscles in their neck to help them breathe. These people may be at greater risk for serious breathing problems with **BOTOX** or **BOTOX Cosmetic**.
- Swallowing problems may last for several months. People who cannot swallow well may need a feeding tube to receive food and water. If swallowing problems are severe, food or liquids may go into your lungs. People who already have swallowing or breathing problems before receiving **BOTOX** or **BOTOX Cosmetic** have the highest risk of getting these problems.

2. Spread of toxin effects. In some cases, the effect of botulinum toxin may affect areas of the body away from the injection site and cause symptoms of a serious condition called botulism. The symptoms of botulism include:
- loss of strength and muscle weakness all over the body
- double vision
- blurred vision and drooping eyelids
- hoarseness or change or loss of voice (dysphonia)
- trouble saying words clearly (dysarthria)
- loss of bladder control
- trouble breathing
- trouble swallowing.

These symptoms can happen hours, days, to weeks after you receive an injection of **BOTOX** or **BOTOX Cosmetic**.

These problems could make it unsafe for you to drive a car or do other dangerous activities. See "What should I avoid while receiving **BOTOX** or **BOTOX Cosmetic**?"

There has not been a confirmed serious case of spread of toxin effect away from the injection site when **BOTOX** has been used at the recommended dose to treat chronic migraine, severe underarm sweating, blepharospasm, or strabismus, or when **BOTOX Cosmetic** has been used at the recommended dose to treat frown lines.

What are BOTOX and BOTOX Cosmetic?

BOTOX is a prescription medicine that is injected into muscles and used:
- to treat overactive bladder symptoms such as a strong need to urinate with leaking or wetting accidents (urge urinary incontinence), a strong need to urinate right away (urgency), and urinating often (frequency) in adults when another type of medicine (anticholinergic) does not work well enough or cannot be taken.
- to treat leakage of urine (incontinence) in adults with overactive bladder due to neurologic disease when another type of medicine (anticholinergic) does not work well enough or cannot be taken.

7

- to prevent headaches in adults with chronic migraine who have 15 or more days each month with headache lasting 4 or more hours each day.
- to treat increased muscle stiffness in elbow, wrist, and finger muscles in adults with upper limb spasticity.
- to treat the abnormal head position and neck pain that happens with cervical dystonia (CD) in adults.
- to treat certain types of eye muscle problems (strabismus) or abnormal spasm of the eyelids (blepharospasm) in people 12 years and older.

BOTOX is also injected into the skin to treat the symptoms of severe underarm sweating (severe primary axillary hyperhidrosis) when medicines used on the skin (topical) do not work well enough.

BOTOX Cosmetic is a prescription medicine that is injected into muscles and used to improve the look of moderate to severe frown lines between the eyebrows (glabellar lines) in adults younger than 65 years of age for a short period of time (temporary).

It is not known whether **BOTOX** is safe or effective in people younger than:
- 18 years of age for treatment of urinary incontinence
- 18 years of age for treatment of chronic migraine
- 18 years of age for treatment of spasticity
- 16 years of age for treatment of cervical dystonia
- 18 years of age for treatment of hyperhidrosis
- 12 years of age for treatment of strabismus or blepharospasm.

BOTOX Cosmetic is not recommended for use in children younger than 18 years of age.

It is not known whether **BOTOX** and **BOTOX Cosmetic** are safe or effective to prevent headaches in people with migraine who have 14 or fewer headache days each month (episodic migraine).

It is not known whether **BOTOX** and **BOTOX Cosmetic** are safe or effective for other types of muscle spasms or for severe sweating anywhere other than your armpits.

Who should not take BOTOX or BOTOX Cosmetic?

Do not take **BOTOX** or **BOTOX Cosmetic** if you:
- are allergic to any of the ingredients in **BOTOX** or **BOTOX Cosmetic**. See the end of this Medication Guide for a list of ingredients in **BOTOX** and **BOTOX Cosmetic**.
- had an allergic reaction to any other botulinum toxin product such as *Myobloc*, *Dysport*, or *Xeomin*
- have a skin infection at the planned injection site – are being treated for urinary incontinence and have a urinary tract infection (UTI) – are being treated for urinary incontinence and find that you cannot empty your bladder on your own (only applies to people who are not routinely catheterizing).

What should I tell my doctor before taking BOTOX or BOTOX Cosmetic? Tell your doctor about all your medical conditions, including if you:
- have a disease that affects your muscles and nerves (such as amyotrophic lateral sclerosis [ALS or Lou Gehrig's disease], myasthenia gravis or Lambert-Eaton syndrome). See "What is the most important information I should know about **BOTOX** and **BOTOX Cosmetic**?"
- have allergies to any botulinum toxin product
- had any side effect from any botulinum toxin product in the past
- have or have had a breathing problem, such as asthma or emphysema
- have or have had swallowing problems
- have or have had bleeding problems
- have plans to have surgery
- had surgery on your face
- have weakness of your forehead muscles, such as trouble raising your eyebrows
- have drooping eyelids
- have any other change in the way your face normally looks
- have symptoms of a urinary tract infection (UTI) and are being treated for urinary incontinence. Symptoms of a urinary tract infection may include pain or burning with urination, frequent urination, or fever.
- have problems emptying your bladder on your own and are being treated for urinary incontinence
- are pregnant or plan to become pregnant. It is not known if **BOTOX** or **BOTOX** Cosmetic can harm your unborn baby.
- are breast-feeding or plan to breastfeed. It is not known if **BOTOX** or **BOTOX** Cosmetic passes into breast milk.

Tell your doctor about all the medicines you take, including prescription and nonprescription medicines, vitamins and herbal products. Using **BOTOX** or **BOTOX Cosmetic** with certain other medicines may cause serious side effects. Do not start any new medicines until you have told your doctor that you have received **BOTOX** or **BOTOX Cosmetic** in the past.

Especially tell your doctor if you:
- have received any other botulinum toxin product in the past 4 months
- have received injections of botulinum toxin, such as Myobloc (rimabotulinumtoxinB), Dysport (abobotulinumtoxinA), or Xeomin (incobotulinumtoxinA) in the past. Be sure your doctor knows exactly which product you received.
- have recently received an antibiotic by injection
- take muscle relaxants
- take an allergy or cold medicine
- take a sleep medicine
- take anti-platelets (aspirin-like products) and/or anti-coagulants (blood thinners).

Ask your doctor if you are not sure if your medicine is one that is listed above.

Know the medicines you take. Keep a list of your medicines with you to show your doctor and pharmacist each time you get a new medicine.

How should I take BOTOX or BOTOX Cosmetic?
- **BOTOX** or **BOTOX Cosmetic** is an injection that your doctor will give you.
- **BOTOX** is injected into your affected muscles, skin, or bladder.
- **BOTOX Cosmetic** is injected into your affected muscles.
- Your doctor may change your dose of **BOTOX** or **BOTOX Cosmetic**, until you and your doctor find the best dose for you.
- Your doctor will tell you how often you will receive your dose of **BOTOX** or **BOTOX Cosmetic** injections.

What should I avoid while taking BOTOX or BOTOX Cosmetic?

BOTOX and **BOTOX Cosmetic** may cause loss of strength or general muscle weakness, or vision problems within hours to weeks of taking **BOTOX** or **BOTOX Cosmetic**. If this happens, do not drive a car, operate machinery, or do other dangerous activities. See "What is the most important information I should know about **BOTOX** and **BOTOX Cosmetic**?"

What are the possible side effects of BOTOX and BOTOX Cosmetic?

BOTOX and **BOTOX Cosmetic** can cause serious side effects. See "What is the most important information I should know about **BOTOX** and **BOTOX** Cosmetic?"

Reference ID: 3247784

Other side effects of BOTOX and BOTOX Cosmetic include:
- dry mouth.
- discomfort or pain at the injection site.
- tiredness.
- headache.
- neck pain.
- eye problems: double vision, blurred vision, decreased eyesight, drooping eyelids, swelling of your eyelids, and dry eyes.
- urinary tract infection in people being treated for urinary incontinence.
- painful urination in people being treated for urinary incontinence.
- inability to empty your bladder on your own and are being treated for urinary incontinence. If you have difficulty fully emptying your bladder after getting **BOTOX**, you may need to use disposable self-catheters to empty your bladder up to a few times each day until your bladder is able to start emptying again.
- allergic reactions. Symptoms of an allergic reaction to **BOTOX** or **BOTOX Cosmetic** may include: itching, rash, red itchy welts, wheezing, asthma symptoms, or dizziness or feeling faint. Tell your doctor or get medical help right away if you are wheezing or have asthma symptoms, or if you become dizzy or faint.

Tell your doctor if you have any side effect that bothers you or that does not go away.

These are not all the possible side effects of **BOTOX** and **BOTOX Cosmetic**. For more information, ask your doctor or pharmacist. Call your doctor for medical advice about side effects. You may report side effects to FDA at 1-800-FDA-1088.

General information about BOTOX and BOTOX Cosmetic:

Medicines are sometimes prescribed for purposes other than those listed in a Medication Guide.

This Medication Guide summarizes the most important information about BOTOX and BOTOX Cosmetic. If you would like more information, talk with your doctor. You can ask your doctor or pharmacist for information about BOTOX and BOTOX Cosmetic that is written for health-care professionals. For more information about BOTOX and BOTOX Cosmetic call Allergan at 1-800-433-8871 or go to www.BOTOX.com.

What are the ingredients in **BOTOX** and **BOTOX Cosmetic**?

Active ingredient: botulinum toxin type A

Inactive ingredients: human albumin and sodium chloride

This Medication Guide has been approved by the U.S. Food and Drug Administration.
Manufactured by: Allergan Pharmaceuticals Ireland a subsidiary of: Allergan, Inc. 2525 Dupont Dr. Irvine, CA 92612
Revised: 01/2013
© 2013 Allergan, Inc.
®-marks owned by Allergan, Inc.
Patented. See: www.allergan.com/products/patent_notices
Myobloc® is a registered trademark of Solstice Neurosciences, Inc.
Dysport® is a registered trademark of Ipsen Biopharm Limited Company.
Xeomin® is a registered trademark of Merz Pharma GmbH & Co KGaA.
Reference ID: 3247784

7

Medication Guide XEOMIN

(Zeo-min)
(incobotulinumtoxinA)
for injection, for intramuscular use

Read this Medication Guide before you start receiving **XEOMIN** and each time **XEOMIN** is given to you. There may be new information. This information does not take the place of talking to your doctor about your medical condition or your treatment. You should share this information with your family members and caregivers.

What is the most important information that I should know about XEOMIN?

XEOMIN may cause serious side effects that can be life threatening. Call your doctor or get medical help right away if you have any of these problems after treatment with XEOMIN:
- **Problems with swallowing, speaking, or breathing. These problems can happen hours to weeks after an injection of XEOMIN** If the muscles that you use to breathe and swallow become weak after the injection. Death can happen as a complication if you have severe problems with swallowing or breathing after treatment with **XEOMIN**.
- People with certain breathing problems may need to use muscles in their neck to help them breathe. These patients may be at greater risk for serious breathing problems with **XEOMIN**.
- Swallowing problems may last for several months. People who cannot swallow well may need a feeding tube to receive food and water. If swallowing problems are severe, food or liquids may go into your lungs. People who already have swallowing or breathing problems before receiving XEOMIN have the highest risk of getting these problems.
- **Spread of toxin effects.** In some cases, the effect of botulinum toxin may affect areas of the body away from the injection site and cause symptoms of a serious condition called botulism. The symptoms of botulism include:
  - loss of strength and muscle weakness all over the body
  - double vision
  - blurred vision and drooping eyelids
  - hoarseness or change or loss of voice
  - trouble saying words clearly
  - loss of bladder control
  - trouble breathing
  - trouble swallowing.

These symptoms can happen hours to weeks after you receive an injection of XEOMIN.

These problems could make it unsafe for you to drive a car or do other dangerous activities. See "What should I avoid while receiving XEOMIN?"

What is XEOMIN?

XEOMIN is a prescription medicine that is injected into muscles and used:
- to treat the abnormal head position and neck pain that happens with cervical dystonia (CD) in adults.
- to treat abnormal spasm of the eyelids (blepharospasm) in adults who have had prior treatment with onabotulinumtoxinA (BOTOX).
- to improve the look of moderate to severe frown lines between the eyebrows (glabellar lines) in adults for a short period of time (temporary).

It is not known whether XEOMIN is safe or effective in children.

Who should not take XEOMIN?

Do not take XEOMIN if you:
- are allergic to XEOMIN or any of the ingredients in XEOMIN. **See the end of this Medication Guide for a list of ingredients in XEOMIN.**
- had an allergic reaction to any other botulinum toxin products such as rimabotulinumtoxinB (MYOBLOC, onabotulinumtoxinA (**BOTOX**, **BOTOX** COSMETIC), or abobotulinumtoxinA (DYSPORT).
- have a skin infection at the planned injection site.

What should I tell my doctor before receiving XEOMIN?

Before you take XEOMIN tell your doctor about all your medical conditions, including if you:
- have a disease that affects your muscles and nerves (such as amyotrophic lateral sclerosis [ALS or Lou Gehrig's disease], myasthenia gravis or Lambert-Eaton syndrome). **See "What is the most important information I should know about XEOMIN?"**
- have allergies to any botulinum toxin product
- have had any side effect from any other botulinum toxin in the past
- have a breathing problem, such as asthma or emphysema
- have a history of swallowing problems or inhaling food or fluid into your lungs (aspiration)
- have bleeding problems
- have drooping eyelids
- have plans to have surgery
- have had surgery on your face
- are pregnant or plan to become pregnant. It is not known if XEOMIN can harm your unborn baby
- are breastfeeding or plan to breastfeed. It is not known if XEOMIN passes into breast milk.

Tell your doctor about all the medicines you take, including prescription and nonprescription medicines, vitamins and herbal supplements.

Using XEOMIN with certain other medicines may cause serious side effects. **Do not start any new medicines until you have told your doctor that you have received XEOMIN in the past**.

Especially tell your doctor if you:
- have received any other botulinum toxin product in the past 4 months
- have received injections of botulinum toxin such as rimabotulinumtoxinB (MYOBLOC, onabotulinumtoxinA (BOTOX, BOTOX COSMETIC) and abobotulinumtoxinA (DYSPORT) in the past. Be sure your doctor knows exactly which product you received. The dose of **XEOMIN** may be different from other botulinum toxin products that you have received
- have recently received an antibiotic by injection
- take muscle relaxants
- take an allergy or cold medicine
- take a sleep medicine
- take a blood thinner medicine.

Ask your doctor if you are not sure if your medicine is one that is listed above.

Know the medicines you take. Keep a list of your medicines with you to show your doctor and pharmacist each time you get a new medicine.

How wil I receive XEOMIN?
- XEOMIN is a shot (injection) that your doctor will give you.
- XEOMIN is injected into your affected muscles.
- Your doctor may change your dose of XEOMIN until you and your doctor find the best dose for you.

What should I avoid while receiving XEOMIN?

XEOMIN may cause loss of strength or general muscle weakness, blurred vision, or drooping eyelids within hours to weeks of taking XEOMIN. **If this happens, do not drive a car, operate machinery, or do other dangerous activities.** See "What is the most important information I should know about XEOMIN?"

What are the possible side effects of XEOMIN?

XEOMIN can cause serious side effects. See "What is the most important information I should know about XEOMIN?"
- **XEOMIN** may cause other serious side effects including allergic reactions. Symptoms of an allergic reaction to XEOMIN may include: itching, rash, redness, swelling, wheezing, asthma symptoms, or dizziness or feeling faint. Tell your doctor or get medical help right away if you get wheezing or asthma symptoms, or if you get dizzy or faint.

The most common side effects of XEOMIN include:
- dry mouth
- discomfort or pain at the injection site
- tiredness

7

- headache
- neck pain
- muscle weakness
- eye problems, including: double vision, blurred vision, drooping eyelids, swelling of your eyelids, and dry eyes. Reduced blinking can also occur. Tell your doctor or get medical help right away if you have eye pain or irritation following treatment.

Tell your doctor if you have any side effect that bothers you or that does not go away.

These are not all the possible side effects of XEOMIN. For more information, ask your doctor or pharmacist.

Call your doctor for medical advice about side effects. You may report side effects to FDA at 1-800-FDA-1088.

General information about XEOMIN

Medicines are sometimes prescribed for purposes other than those listed in a Medication Guide.

XEOMIN should not be used for a condition for which it was not prescribed.

This Medication Guide summarizes the most important information about XEOMIN. If you would like more information, talk with your doctor. You can ask your doctor or pharmacist for information about XEOMIN that is written for healthcare professionals.

For more information go to www.Xeomin.com or call 888-493-6646.

What are the ingredients in XEOMIN?

Active ingredient: incobotulinumtoxinA

Inactive ingredients: human albumin and sucrose

Distributed by: Merz Pharmaceuticals, LLC
4215 Tudor Lane
Greensboro, NC 27410

and

Merz Aesthetics, Inc.
4133 Courtney Road, Suite 10
Franksville, WI 53126

This Medication Guide has been approved by the U.S. Food and Drug Administration.
Issued 07/2011
© 2011 Merz Pharmaceuticals, LLC
XEOMIN® isa registered trademark of Merz Pharma GmbH & Co KGaA. Patent pending.
Botox®, Botox® Cosmetic, Dysport®, and Myobloc® are registered trademarks of their respective owners.

MEDICATION GUIDE DYSPORT

(DIS-port)
(abobotulinumtoxin A)
Injection

Read the Medication Guide that comes with DYSPORT before you start using it and each time DYSPORT is given to you. There may be new information. This information does not take the place of talking with your doctor about your medical condition or your treatment. You should share this information with your family members and caregivers.

What is the most important information I should know about DYSPORT?

DYSPORT may cause serious side effects that can be life threatening including:
- **Problems breathing or swallowing**
- **Spread of toxin effects.**

These problems can happen within hours, or days to weeks after an injection of DYSPORT. Call your doctor or get medical help right away if you have any of these problems after treatment with DYSPORT:

1. Problems swallowing, speaking, or breathing. These problems can happen within hours, or days to weeks after an injection of DYSPORT, usually because the muscles that you use to breathe and swallow can become weak after the injection. Death can happen as a complication if you have severe problems with swallowing or breathing after treatment with DYSPORT.
- People with certain breathing problems may need to use muscles in their neck to help them breathe. These patients may be at greater risk for serious breathing problems with DYSPORT.
- Swallowing problems may last for several weeks. People who can not swallow well may need a feeding tube to receive food and water. If swallowing problems are severe, food or liquids may go into your lungs. People who already have swallowing or breathing problems before receiving DYSPORT have the highest risk of getting these problems.

2. Spread of toxin effects. In some cases, the effect of botulinum toxin may affect areas of the body away from the injection site and cause symptoms of a serious condition called botulism. The symptoms of botulism include:
- loss of strength and muscle weakness all over the body
- double vision
- blurred vision and drooping eyelids
- hoarseness or change or loss of voice (dysphonia)
- trouble saying words clearly (dysarthria)
- loss of bladder control
- trouble breathing
- trouble swallowing.

These symptoms can happen within hours, or days to weeks after you receive an injection of DYSPORT.

These problems could make it unsafe for you to drive a car or do other dangerous activities. See "What should I avoid while receiving DYSPORT?"

What is DYSPORT?

DYSPORT is a prescription medicine that is injected into muscles and used:
- to treat the abnormal head position and neck pain that happens with cervical dystonia (CD) in adults
- to improve the look of moderate to severe frown lines between the eyebrows (glabellar lines) in adults younger than 65 years of age for a short period of time (temporary).

CD is caused by muscle spasms in the neck. These spasms cause abnormal position of the head and often neck pain. After DYSPORT is injected into muscles, those muscles are weakened for up to 12 to 16 weeks or longer. This may help lessen your symptoms.

Frown lines (wrinkles) happen because the muscles that control facial expression are used often (muscle tightening over and over). After DYSPORT is injected into the muscles that control facial expression, the medicine stops the tightening of these muscles for up to 4 months.

It is not known whether DYSPORT is safe or effective in children under 18 years of age.

7

It is not known whether DYSPORT is safe or effective for the treatment of other types of muscle spasms. It is not known whether DYSPORT is safe or effective for the treatment of other wrinkles.

Who should not take DYSPORT?

Do not take DYSPORT if you:
- are allergic to DYSPORT or any of the ingredients in DYSPORT. See the end of this Medication Guide for a list of ingredients in DYSPORT
- are allergic to cow's milk protein
- had an allergic reaction to any other botulinum toxin product such as Myobloc (rimabotulinumtoxinB)*, Botox (onabotulinumtoxinA)*, or Xeomin (incobotulinumtoxinA)*
- have a skin infection at the planned injection site.

What should I tell my doctor before taking DYSPORT?

Tell your doctor about all your medical conditions, including if you:
- have a disease that affects your muscles and nerves (such as amyotrophic lateral sclerosis [ALS or Lou Gehrig's disease], myasthenia gravis or Lambert-Eaton syndrome). See "What is the most important information I should know about DYSPORT?"
- have allergies to any botulinum toxin product
- had any side effect from any botulinum toxin product in the past
- have or have had a breathing problem, such as asthma or emphysema
- have or have had swallowing problems
- have or have had bleeding problems
- have diabetes
- have or have had a slow heart beat or other problem with your heart rate or rhythm
- have plans to have surgery
- had surgery on your face
- have weakness of your forehead muscles (such as trouble raising your eyebrows)
- have drooping eyelids
- have any other change in the way your face normally looks
- are pregnant or plan to become pregnant. It is not known if **DYSPORT** can harm your unborn baby
- are breast-feeding or planning to breast-feed. It is not known if **DYSPORT** passes into breast milk.

Tell your doctor about all the medicines you take, including prescription and nonprescription medicines, vitamins and herbal products. Using DYSPORT with certain other medicines may cause serious side effects. **Do not start any new medicines until you have told your doctor that you have received DYSPORT in the past.**

Especially tell your doctor if you:
- have received any other botulinum toxin product in the past 4months
- have received injections of botulinum toxin, such as Myobloc (rimabotulinumtoxinB), Botox (onabotulinumtoxinA) or Xeomin (incobotulinumtoxinA) in the past; be sure your doctor knows exactly which product you received
- have recently received an antibiotic by injection
- take muscle relaxants
- take an allergy or cold medicine
- take a sleep medicine.

Ask your doctor if you are not sure if your medicine is one that is listed above.

Know the medicines you take. Keep a list of your medicines with you to show your doctor and pharmacist each time you get a new medicine.

How should I take DYSPORT?
- DYSPORT is an injection that your doctor will give you.
- DYSPORT is injected into the affected muscles.
- Your doctor may give you another dose of DYSPORT after 12 weeks or longer, if it is needed.
- If you are being treated for CD, your doctor may change your dose of DYSPORT, until you and your doctor find the best dose for you.
- The dose of DYSPORT is not the same as the dose of any other botulinum toxin product.

---

*   All trademarks are the property of their respective owners.

What should I avoid while taking DYSPORT?

DYSPORT may cause loss of strength or general muscle weakness, blurred vision, or drooping eyelids within hours to weeks of taking DYS-PORT. **If this happens, do not drive a car, operate machinery, or do other dangerous activities. See "What is the most important information I should know about DYSPORT?"**

What are the possible side effects of DYSPORT?

DYSPORT can cause serious side effects. See "What is the most important information I should know about DYSPORT?"

Other side effects of DYSPORT include:
- dry mouth
- injection site discomfort or pain
- tiredness
- headache
- neck pain
- muscle pain
- eye problems: double vision, blurred vision, decreased eyesight, problems with focusing the eyes (accommodation), drooping eyelids, swelling of the eyelids
- allergic reactions. Symptoms of an allergic reaction to DYSPORT may include: itching, rash, red itchy welts, wheezing, asthma symptoms, or dizziness or feeling faint. Tell your doctor or get medical help right away if you get wheezing or asthma symptoms, or if you get dizzy or faint.

Tell your doctor if you have any side effect that bothers you or that does not go away. These are not all the possible side effects of DYSPORT. For more information, ask your doctor or pharmacist.

Call your doctor for medical advice about side effects. You may report side effects to FDA at 1–800–FDA–1088. General information about DYSPORT:

Medicines are sometimes prescribed for purposes other than those listed in a Medication Guide.

This Medication Guide summarizes the most important information about DYSPORT. If you would like more information, talk with your doctor. You can ask your doctor or pharmacist for information about DYSPORT that is written for healthcare professionals. For more information about DYSPORT call 877-397-7671 or go to www.dysport.com or www.DysportUSA.com.

What are the ingredients in DYSPORT?

Active ingredient: (botulinum toxin Type A)

Inactive ingredients: human albumin, and lactose. DYSPORT may contain cow's milk protein.

Revised: MAY 2012

This Medication Guide has been approved by the U.S. Food and Drug Administration.

Distributed by:
Tercica, Inc.
a subsidiary of the Ipsen Group
Brisbane, CA 94005

and

Medicis Aesthetics Inc.
a wholly owned subsidiary of Medicis Pharmaceutical Corporation
Scottsdale, AZ 85256

Reference ID: 3132426

8 **Appendix**

Web adresses

www.botulinum.at (Austrian Dystonia and Botulinum Toxin Working Group)
www.botulinumtoxin.de (Work Group Botulinum Toxin, registered association, German Society for Neurology)
www.botox.com
www.xeomin.com
www.dysport.com
www.bocouture.com
www.galderma.com (information about Azzalure)
www.allergan.com (information about Botox and Vistabel)
www.myobloc.com
www.neurobloc.info
www.fda.gov
www.ema.europa.eu (European Medecines Agency)
www.dgbt.de (German Society for Aesthetic Botulinum Toxin Therapy)
www.dgn.org (German Society for Neurology, registered association)
www.dystonie.de (German Dystonia Society, registered association)
www.neurotoxininstitute.org/de (The Neuron Toxine Institute, New York)
www.vdaepc.de (Association of German Aesthetic Plastic Surgeons)
www.gacd.de (Society for Aesthetic Surgery Germany, registered association)
www.dgaepc.de (German Society for Aesthetic Plastic Surgery)
www.dgaed.de (German Society for Aesthetic Dermatology)
http://www.plasticsurgery.org/ (American Society of Plastic Surgeons)
http://www.surgery.org/ (American Society for Aesthetic Plastic Surgery)

8

List of videos

Title	Book page	QR-Code	URL
Examination and functional testing	25		http://www.kvm-tv.de/BTX/btx001.mp4
Basic hand position	33		http://www.kvm-tv.de/BTX/btx003.mp4
Basic rules of injection	33		http://www.kvm-tv.de/BTX/btx004.mp4
Rules for safe injecting	35		http://www.kvm-tv.de/BTX/btx005.mp4
Direct injection technique	36		http://www.kvm-tv.de/BTX/btx006.mp4
Directed injection technique	37		http://www.kvm-tv.de/BTX/btx007.mp4
Two-level injection technique	38		http://www.kvm-tv.de/BTX/btx008.mp4

Title	Book page	QR-Code	URL
Subdermal wheal technique	40		http://www.kvm-tv.de/BTX/btx009.mp4
Marking	41		http://www.kvm-tv.de/BTX/btx010.mp4
Treatment of horizontal lines on the forehead	46–49		http://www.kvm-tv.de/BTX/btx011.mp4
Treatment of glabella lines	50–53		http://www.kvm-tv.de/BTX/btx012.mp4
Chemical brow lift	56–58		http://www.kvm-tv.de/BTX/btx013.mp4
Top third of the face- Case 1	130–131		http://www.kvm-tv.de/BTX/btx014.mp4
Top third of the face- Case 2	132–133		http://www.kvm-tv.de/BTX/btx015.mp4
Top third of the face- Case 3	134–135		http://www.kvm-tv.de/BTX/btx016.mp4
Top third of the face- Case 4	136–137		http://www.kvm-tv.de/BTX/btx017.mp4
Top third of the face- Case 5	138–139		http://www.kvm-tv.de/BTX/btx018.mp4

Image sources

Pp. 3, 4, 143-153: Merz Pharmaceuticals GmbH, Frankfurt/Main, Germany
P. 13: Canon Deutschland GmbH, Krefeld, Germany
Pp. 106-139: Archive Dr. G. Sattler, Darmstadt, Germany

Manufacturer directory

Omnican 0.30 × 8 mm, single use insulin syringe with integrated needle: B Braun, Melsungen, Germany
1 ml Luer-Lok Syringe, syringes: BD, Franklin Lakes, USA
Micro-Fine 0.30 × 8 mm, insulin syringes: BD, Franklin Lakes, USA
Microlance 0.30 × 13 mm, needles: BD, Franklin Lakes, USA
Steriject 0.25 × 13 mm, needles: TSK, Tochigi, Japan
Emla cream, AstraZeneca GmbH, Germany

Bibliography

Ascher B. Injection Treatments in Cosmetic Surgery. London: Informa Healthcare, 2008.

Benninghoff A. Anatomie – Makroskopische Anatomie, Embryologie und Histologie des Menschen, vol 1. Munich: Urban & Schwarzenberg, 1994.

Binz T et al. Cell entry strategy of botulinum neurotoxins. Lavoisier: Rencontres en toxinologie, 2007.

Bluemel J, Frevert J, Schwaier A. Comparative Autigenicity of Three Preparations of Botulinum Neurotoxin Type A in the Rabbit. Neurotox Res 2006;9(2):60.

Carruthers A, Carruthers J. Procedures in Cosmetic Dermatology – Botulinum Toxin, ed 2. Philadelphia: Saunders, 2008.

Carruthers A et al. A Validated Brow Positioning Grading Scale. Dermatol Surg 2008;34:150-154.

Carruthers A et al. A Validated Hand Grading Scale. Dermatol Surg 2008;34:179-183.

Carruthers A et al. A Validated Lip Fullness Grading Scale. Dermatol Surg 2008;34:161-166.

Carruthers A et al. A Validated Grading Scale for Crow's Feet. Dermatol Surg 2008;34:173-178.

Carruthers A et al. A Validated Grading Scale for Forehead Lines. Dermatol Surg 2008;34:155-160.

Carruthers A et al. A Validated Grading Scale for Marionette Lines. Dermatol Surg 2008;34:167-172.

Chai Q et al. Structural basis of cell surface receptor recognition by botulinum neurotoxin B. Nature Letters 2006;05411.3d.

Clarijs JP et al. Compendium topografische en kinesiologische Ontleekunde. Vrije Universiteit Brussel (in press).

Cody J. Visualizing muscles – A new ecorche approach to surface anatomy. Lawrence: University press of Kansas KS, 1990.

Dong M et al. SV2 Is the Protein Receptor for Botulinum Neurotoxin A. Science 2006;312:592-596.

Dressler D et al. Equivalent potency of Xeomin® and Botox®. Movement Disorders 2008;23(1, suppl).

Dressler D. Klinische Relevanz von Botulinum-Toxin-Antikörpern. Der Nervenarzt 2008;79(1, suppl):36-40.

Field D. Anatomy – Palpation & surface markings, ed 2. Oxford: Butterworth-Heinemann, 1997.

Foster KA, Bigalke H, Aoki KR. Botulinum Neurotoxin – From Laboratory to Bedside. Neurotoxicity Research 2006;9(2, 3):133-140.

Fritsch C. Wirksamkeit des neuen, komplexprotein-freien Botulinumtoxins (Xeomin®) in der Therapie mimischer Lachfalten. Kosmetische Medizin 2006;27(3) (special issue).

Geiringer SR. Elektromyographie. Atlas zur präzisen Muskellokalisation. Ulm, Stuttgart, Jena, Lübeck: Gustav Fischer, 1997.

Giess R, Werner E, Beck M et al. Impaired salivary gland function reveals autonomic dysfunction in amyotrophic lateral sclerosis. J Neurol 2002;249:1246-1249.

Heckmann M, Ceballos-Baumann AO, Plewig G. Botulinum toxin for axillary hyperhidrosis (excessive sweating). N Engl J Med 2001;344:488-493.

Heckmann M, Rzany B. Botulinumtoxin in der Dermatologie – Grundlagen und praktische Anwendung. München: Urban und Vogel, 2002.

Jost WH. Bildatlas der Botulinumtoxin-Injektion, ed 2. Marburg: KVM, 2009.

Jost WH, Bluemel J, Grafe S. Botulinum Neurotoxin Type A Free of Complexing Proteins (Xeomin®) in Focal Dystonia. Drugs 2007;67(5):669-683.

Jost WH. Efficacy and safety of botulinum neurotoxin type A free of complexing proteins (NT 201) in cervical dystonia and blepharospasm. Future Neurol. 2007;2(5):485-493.

Jost WH, Kohl A. Botulinum toxin: evidence-based medicine criteria in rare indications. J Neurol 2001;248(1, suppl):39-44.

Khorram R. Faltentherapie mit einem neuen komplexproteinfreien Botulinumtoxin A (Xeomin®) bei 40 Patienten. Ästhetische Dermatologie 2007 (special issue).

Leonhardt H, Tillmann B, Töndury G, Zilles K. Rauber/Kopsch, Anatomie des Menschen, 4 volumes. New York: Thieme, 1998.

Maack M et al. Botulinumtoxin A – Beeinflussen Komplexproteine das Diffusionsverhalten? Der Deutsche Dermatologe 2007;55(8):562-563.

Mahrhold S et al. The synaptic vesicle protein 2C mediates the uptake of botulinum neurotoxin A into phrenic nerves. FEBS Letters 2006;580:2011-2014.

De Maio M, Rzany B. Botulinum Toxin in Aesthetic Medicine. Berlin: Springer, 2007.

Münchau A, Bhatia KP. Clinical review: Use of botulinum toxin injection in medicine today. BMJ 2000;320:161-165.

Palastanga N, Field D, Soames R. Anatomy and human movement. ed 4. Oxford: Butterworth-Heinemann, 2002.

Palmar Saadia D, Voustianiouk A, Wang AK et al. Botulinum toxin type A in primary palmar hyperhidrosis: randomized, single-blind, two-dose study. Neurology 2001;57:2095-2099.

Platzer W. Taschenatlas Anatomie. Vol 1: Bewegungsapparat. ed 9. Stuttgart: Thieme, 2005.

Prager W et al. Wirksamkeit und Verträglichkeit des neuen, komplexprotein-freien Botulinumtoxins (Xeomin®) bei der Behandlung von mimischen Falten – Untersuchungsergebnisse. Kosmetische Medizin 2007;2 (special issue).

Roggenkämper P et al. Efficacy and safety of a new Botulinum Toxin Type A free of complexing proteins in the treatment of blepharospasm. J Neural Transm 2006;113:303-312.

Rongsheng J et al. Botulinum neurotoxin B regonizes its protein receptor with high affinity and specificity. Nature 2006;444(21):1092-1095.

Rummel A et al. Synaptotagmins I and II Act as Nerve Cell Receptors for Botulinum Neurotoxin G. The Journal of Biological Chemistry 2004;279(29):30865-30870.

Schleyer V, Berneburg M. Wirksamkeit und Sicherheit von Botulinum Neurotoxin Typ A (Xeomin®) in der Behandlung der Glabellafalte. Kosmetische Medizin 2008;29(3) (special issue).

Schmitt A, Dreyer F, John C. At Least Three Sequential Steps are Involved in the Tetanus Toxin-Induced Block of Neuromuscular Transmission. Naunyn-Schmiedeberg's Arch Pharmacol 1981;317:326-330.

Schünke M, Schulte E, Schumacher U et al. Prometheus LernAtlas der Anatomie – Kopf und Neuroanatomie. Stuttgart, New York: Thieme, 2006.

Sobotta J. Atlas der Anatomie des Menschen, vol 1 & 2. Munich: Urban & Fischer, 2000.

Sommer B, Sattler G (eds). Botulinumtoxin in der ästhetischen Medizin, ed 3. Stuttgart, New York: Thieme, 2006.

Terminologia Anatomica. Stuttgart: Thieme, 1998.

Valerius KP, Frank A, Kolster BC. Das Muskelbuch. Anatomie, Untersuchung, Bewegung, ed 3. Marburg: KVM, 2007.

8

Index

8

8

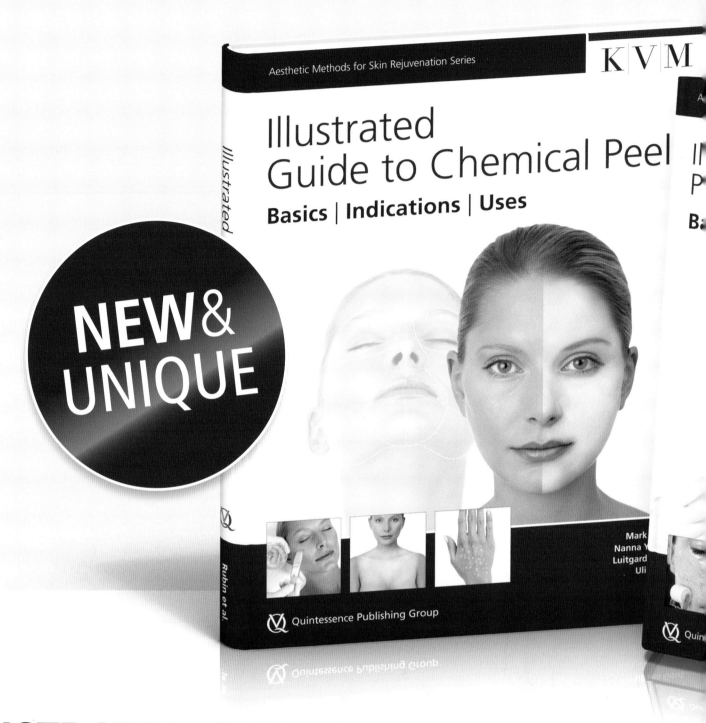

On the book cover:

ILLUSTRATED GUIDES
TO TECHNIQUES IN AESTHETIC MEDICINE

Forthcoming in the Aesthetic Methods for Skin Rejuvenation Series:

Illustrated Guide to Chemical Peels, Illustrated Guide to Percutaneous Collagen Induction &
Illustrated Guide to Injectable Fillers. More information available at www.quintpub.co.uk or at www.quintpub.com

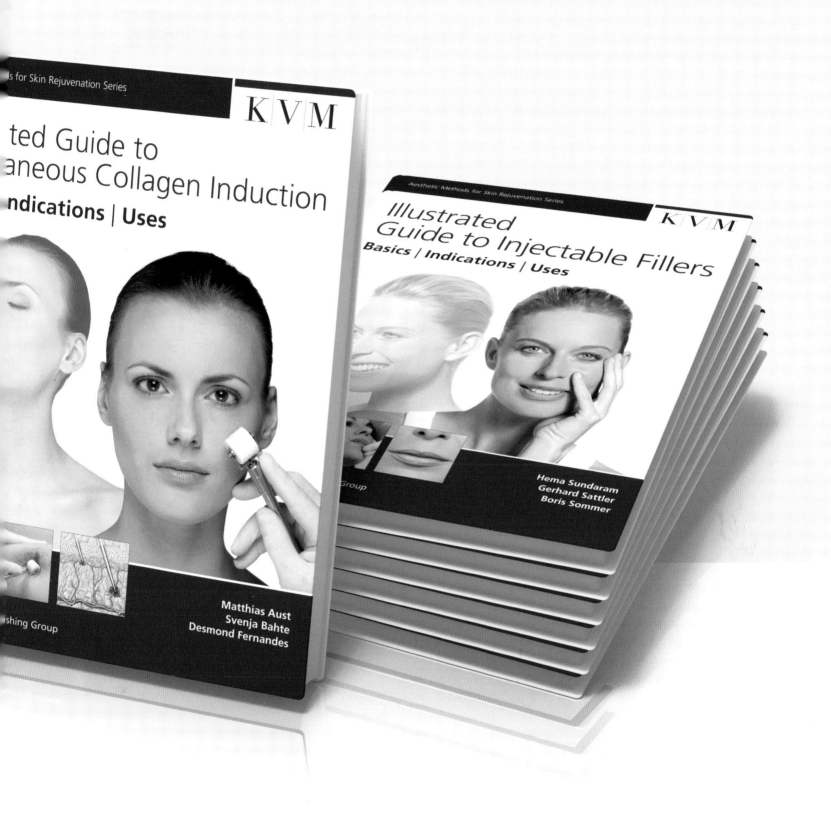